GROWING HERBAL MEDICINE AT HOME FOR BEGINNERS

A Step-By-Step Guide To Planting, Harvesting, And Using Medicinal Herbs For Natural Health And Wellness

TABLE OF CONTENTS

Chapter 7: Using Medicinal Herbs for Health and Wellness

7.1 Herbal Remedies for Common Ailments

7.2 Recipes for Herbal Salves and Balms

7.3 Creating Your Own Herbal First Aid Kit

7.4 Incorporating Herbs into Daily Life

Chapter 8: Advanced Herbal Gardening Techniques

8.1 Propagation Methods: Cuttings and Divisions

8.2 Growing Herbs in Containers

8.3 Designing a Medicinal Herb Garden

8.4 Companion Planting Strategies

Chapter 9: Troubleshooting Common Issues

9.1 Identifying and Solving Common Problems

9.2 Dealing with Pests and Diseases

9.3 Soil Health and Fertility Issues

9.4 Seasonal Challenges and Solutions

INTRODUCTION TO HERBAL MEDICINE

Welcome to the realm of herbal medicine. For ages, people have relied on nature's medicine to mend wounds, alleviate afflictions, and stay healthy. Growing your own medicinal herbs is a rewarding activity that ties you to the soil while also providing a sustainable source of natural cures. In this chapter, we'll look at the rich history of herbal medicine, the numerous advantages of growing your own herbs, the fundamental features of medicinal plants, and the necessary safety precautions to use herbs successfully and responsibly.

THE HISTORY OF HERBAL MEDICINE

Herbal medicine is one of the most ancient types of treatment in human history, extending back thousands of years.

- Ancient Civilizations: The Ancient Egyptians, Chinese, Greeks, and Romans all used plants for therapeutic purposes. The Egyptian Ebers Papyrus, written approximately 1550 BC, contains hundreds of herbal medicines.
• Traditional Chinese Medicine (TCM): TCM is over 2,000 years old and relies largely Chinese herbs for healing. The ancient manuscript "Shennong Ben Cao Jing" lists more than 365 therapeutic herbs.
- Ayurveda: Ayurveda, which originated in India,

relies on herbs as a foundation for its comprehensive approach to health, focusing on balance and prevention.
- Native American Practices: Indigenous communities in North America have traditionally employed local plants for medical purposes, with knowledge passed down through generations.

These historical methods paved the way for current herbal treatment, which is becoming increasingly popular as people seek natural alternatives to drugs.

BENEFITS OF GROWING YOUR OWN MEDICAL HERBS

Growing your own medicinal herbs provides numerous advantages that go beyond simple health benefits.

- Self-Sufficiency: Growing your own herbs provides a consistent source of fresh, organic plants for your home apothecary.
- Cost-Effective: Herbal treatments can be expensive to buy, but cultivating your own herbs considerably lowers prices.
- Sustainability: Home gardening reduces your carbon footprint by eliminating the need for transportation and packaging that comes with store-bought herbs.
- Quality Control: You have complete control over

the growing environment, so your herbs will be free of pesticides and other hazardous substances.
- Therapeutic Benefits: Gardening is a stress-relieving and mental-health-promoting pastime.

For example, growing a tiny patch of lavender in your garden can give you with a natural solution for anxiety and insomnia, as well as improve the beauty and aroma of your outdoor environment.

UNDERSTANDING HERBAL PROPERTIES.

To use medical herbs properly, one must first grasp their fundamental qualities and how they interact with the body.

- Active Constituents: These are the chemical substances responsible for a herb's therapeutic properties. For example, peppermint's essential oils contain antispasmodic and digestive effects.
- Herbal actions: Herbs are classed according to their activities, which include anti-inflammatory, antibacterial, diuretic, and sedative. Chamomile is well-known for its soothing and anti-inflammatory effects.
- Synergy: Herbs frequently operate best when combined in ways that make the whole greater than the sum of its parts. This synergistic effect can boost the therapeutic efficacy of herbal treatments.

Understanding these features enables you to formulate successful herbal remedies based on your unique requirements. For example, combining ginger and turmeric can result in an effective anti-inflammatory tea.

SAFETY AND PRECAUTIONS

Herbs are natural, but they are not without risk. It's critical to utilize them responsibly and safely.

- Proper Identification: Before using any plant, always check that it is correctly identified. Some plants have harmful lookalikes.
- Dosage and Preparation: Use the specified doses and preparation techniques. Too much of a herb might be toxic, while too little can be ineffectual.
- Allergies and sensitivities: Be mindful of any potential allergies. To rule out any bad responses, test new herbs in modest amounts.
- Interactions with drugs: Certain herbs may interfere with prescription drugs. Before mixing herbal medicines and conventional treatments, consult a healthcare practitioner.
- Pregnancy and breastfeeding: Some herbs are not suitable for pregnant or breastfeeding women. Always conduct research or consult with a professional before using.

For example, while St. John's Wort is useful for

mild depression, it can interact with birth control pills and other pharmaceuticals, emphasising the significance of recognizing herb-drug interactions.

Growing and using therapeutic herbs brings up new possibilities for natural healing and self-sufficiency. By appreciating the rich history of herbal medicine, recognizing the benefits of growing your own herbs, understanding their qualities, and following safety procedures, you can lay the groundwork for a healthy herbal practice. Whether you're a beginner gardener or a seasoned herbalist, this guide will help you every step of the way as you discover the healing power of nature.

GETTING STARTED WITH HERBAL GARDENING

Herbal gardening is a wonderful activity that connects you with nature while also providing a plentiful supply of therapeutic plants. With proper planning and care, you can grow a thriving herb garden in your backyard or on a small balcony. In this chapter, we'll look at the most important initial step: determining the best location for your herbal garden. Where and how you grow your herbs will have a significant impact on their success. We'll look at essential aspects like sunlight, soil quality, water access, and area needs to guarantee your garden thrives.

CHOOSING THE RIGHT LOCATION

Choosing the best location for your herbal garden requires various factors. A well-chosen location ensures that your herbs have the proper conditions to develop, resulting in a healthy and fruitful garden.

Sunlight Requirements

Most medicinal herbs need plenty of sunlight to become robust and potent.

- Full Sun: Most herbs, including basil, rosemary, and thyme, require at least 6-8 hours of direct

sunlight every day. These plants love the sun and will thrive in a south-facing garden or balcony.
- Partial Shade: Some herbs, such as mint, parsley, and chives, thrive in partial shade, particularly in hot areas. They benefit from morning sunlight and midday shade.
- Indoor Growth: If your outdoor space is limited, consider growing herbs indoors on a sunny windowsill or under grow lights. Herbs like basil, cilantro, and dill thrive in indoor situations.

Example: In a backyard garden, planting your herbs in a sunny location ensures that they receive enough light, yet a strategically placed shade cloth can shelter them from the heavy afternoon heat.

Soil Quality

A productive herbal garden requires healthy soil.

- Well-Draining Soil: Herbs typically dislike soggy soil. To improve soil structure, add organic matter such as compost or sand to ensure proper drainage in your garden.
- pH Levels: Most herbs require slightly acidic or neutral soil (pH 6.0-7.0). Test the pH of your soil and add lime to boost it or sulfur to lower it as needed.
- Fertility of the Soil To provide critical nutrients to your soil, mix in organic compost or well-rotted

manure. Avoid applying chemical fertilizers, as they can harm vital soil bacteria.

Example: A raised bed packed with garden soil, compost, and sand provides a great setting for Mediterranean herbs such as lavender and oregano, which flourish in well-drained soil.

Water Access

Watering your herb garden on a consistent and proper basis is critical to its success.

- Proximity to Water Source: Select a position near a water source for convenient access. This convenience is especially beneficial during dry spells or hot summer months.
- Watering Needs: Group plants that require similar amounts of water together. Drought-tolerant herbs, such as sage and thyme, can be grown together, however moisture-loving plants, such as mint and basil, should be planted separately.
- Irrigation Systems: Install a drip irrigation system or soaker hoses to ensure continuous moisture without overwatering. Mulching around plants also helps to preserve soil moisture.

Example: Planting water-intensive herbs near your garden hose or rain barrel ensures that they receive the necessary frequent watering without exerting too much effort.

Space and Layout

Maximizing available area and designing an efficient layout are essential for a productive herb garden.

- Garden Size Determine your available space and plan accordingly. A modest balcony or windowsill can support a container herb plant.
- Container Gardening: If you have limited ground space, grow herbs in pots, hanging baskets, or vertical planters. Choose containers that have good drainage and enough depth for root growth.
- Garden Beds: Raised or classic in-ground beds are suitable for bigger gardens. Plan pathways that will allow for easy planting, weeding, and harvesting.

Example: A vertical garden on a sunny balcony can grow a variety of herbs such as basil, oregano, and thyme, saving space while adding greenery to your living space.

Choosing the ideal site for your herbal garden establishes the foundation for a vibrant, productive landscape full with therapeutic plants. By taking into account sunshine, soil quality, water availability, and space requirements, you can create an environment in which your herbs can thrive.

Whether you're planting in a large yard or a little balcony, careful planning will ensure that your herbal garden brings you joy, health, and natural treatments.

ESSENTIAL GARDENING TOOLS

Beginning the path of herbal gardening takes not only enthusiasm and knowledge, but also the proper tools. Having the right tools can make gardening jobs more effective, pleasurable, and successful. Whether you're growing in a large backyard or a little balcony, having the right tools will help you grow a healthy and fruitful herb garden. In this section, we'll look at the essential gardening tools that any herbal gardener should have, as well as how to choose and use them properly.

Basic Gardening Tools

Hand Trowel.

A hand trowel is a compact, handheld instrument with a pointed, scoop-shaped metal blade. It's ideal for digging small holes, transplanting plants, and pulling weeds.

- Usage: Perfect for growing herbs in containers or garden beds. Use it to scrape soil, mix in compost, and remove tenacious weeds.

- Here's an example: When planting basil seedlings, use a hand trowel to dig accurate holes and carefully drop the tiny plants into the dirt.

Pruning Shears

Trimming and collecting herbs requires the use of pruning shears, often known as secateurs. They have keen blades capable of cutting through stems and branches cleanly.

- Usage: Use pruning shears to remove dead or damaged leaves, shape plants, and harvest herbs without causing damage to the plant.
- Example: Regularly cutting your mint plants with pruning shears promotes bushier growth and keeps them from getting lanky.

Garden Gloves

Garden gloves protect your hands from dirt, thorns, and blisters while improving your grasp on equipment.

- Usage: Wear gloves to keep your hands clean and safe when planting, gardening, or handling abrasive materials.
- Example: Garden gloves are useful for handling thorny herbs like rosemary to avoid scrapes and skin irritation.

Watering Can

A watering can with a large spout allows you to water your herbs gently and precisely while minimizing soil disturbance.

- Utilization: Choose a can with a replaceable rose (spout attachment) for a variety of watering options, ranging from a delicate sprinkle to a steady stream.
- Here's an example: A watering can with a fine rose is ideal for watering fragile seedlings without removing the soil.

Advanced Gardening Tools

Garden Fork

A garden fork, often called a digging fork or spading fork, is used to remove soil, turn compost, and aerate garden beds.

- Usage: Its robust tines easily penetrate the soil, making it great for loosening compacted soil and incorporating organic matter.
- Example: Before planting a fresh herb bed, loosen the soil with a garden fork and add compost to create a nutrient-rich growing environment.

Hoe

A hoe is a useful implement for weeding, cultivating soil, and making furrows for planting seeds.

- Usage: Use a hoe to remove weeds at the soil level, cultivate the soil surface, and create rows for direct sowing.
- Example: A Dutch hoe with a sharp blade helps you to quickly cut through weeds while without harming neighboring flora.

Garden Rake

A garden rake may help you level the soil, remove debris, and provide a smooth, even area for planting.

- Usage: Use a rake to prepare garden beds, spread mulch, and collect fallen leaves or garden garbage.
- Here's an example: After tilling the soil with a garden fork, use a rake to produce a flat, even area for planting.

Specialized Gardening Tools

Seed Trays and Starter Pots

Seed trays and starter pots are necessary for germinating seeds and nurturing seedlings indoors before transferring them into the garden.

- Usage: Fill trays or pots with seed-starting mix, plant seeds, and offer continuous moisture and temperature to promote germination.
- Here's an example: Using seed trays, you may start a number of herbs indoors, including basil, cilantro, and dill, to ensure strong, healthy seedlings for transplanting.

Plant Markers

Plant markers let you keep track of different herbs, which is especially useful in a diverse garden with several species.

- Usage: Label each herb with its name and planting date to track development and manage your garden more effectively.
- Here's an example: Wooden or plastic signs with herb names such as thyme, sage, and oregano can help you identify plants and remember their special care requirements.

Garden cart or wheelbarrow

A garden cart or wheelbarrow is extremely useful for moving soil, compost, plants, and tools throughout the garden.

- Usage: Use it to conveniently transport heavy loads, reducing physical strain and saving time.

- Here's an example: When mulching your herb garden, a wheelbarrow can assist you transfer huge amounts of mulch from your compost pile to the garden beds quickly.

Equipping yourself with the proper gardening tools is critical for growing a successful and joyful herbal garden. From hand trowels and pruning shears to garden forks and wheelbarrows, each tool is essential for keeping a healthy and productive garden. By selecting high-quality, long-lasting tools and using them correctly, you'll set yourself up for a joyful gardening experience in which your medicinal herbs grow and flourish.

SOIL PREPARATION AND AMENDMENTS

The soil serves as the foundation for any healthy herb garden. Proper soil preparation and amendments are essential for giving your medicinal herbs the nutrition, drainage, and structure they require to grow strong and healthy. In this section, we will look at the importance of soil health, how to prepare your garden bed or containers, and what amendments you can use to improve the quality of your soil. By learning and adopting these techniques, you may create an ideal environment for your herbs to thrive.

Understanding Soil Health.

Healthy soil is brimming with life and provides optimal circumstances for plant growth.

- Soil Composition: Soil consists of minerals, organic materials, water, and air. The balance of these components influences the soil's texture, structure, and fertility.
- Soil Microbes: Beneficial microorganisms such as bacteria, fungi, and earthworms help break down organic debris and release nutrients that plants can consume.
- pH Level: The acidity or alkalinity of your soil (as measured by pH) influences nutrient availability. Most herbs require a pH range of slightly acidic to neutral (6.0-7.0).

Example: Test your soil to establish its composition and pH. This knowledge will help you make informed amendment choices to establish a balanced and fertile growing medium.

Soil Preparation

There are various procedures to preparing your soil so that it suits the needs of your herbs.

Clearing and Tilling

- Remove Weeds and Debris: Make sure the space is

free of weeds, rocks, and other debris that may impede plant growth.

- Tilling Soil: Using a garden fork or tiller, turn the soil to a depth of at least 8 to 12 inches. This loosens the soil, promotes aeration, and allows roots to penetrate more easily.

Example: In a fresh garden bed, use a spade or tiller to break up compacted soil and add organic matter, ensuring a well-aerated and rich planting base.

Adding Organic Matter

- Compost: Adding compost boosts soil structure, fertility, and moisture retention. Spread a 2-3 inch layer of compost over the soil and stir thoroughly.
- Aged Manure: Well-rotted manure replenishes the soil with nutrients. Apply it similarly to compost, making sure it is completely digested to avoid scorching plant roots.
- The Leaf Mold: Decomposed leaves increase organic matter and enhance soil texture. Incorporate it into the soil to increase its water-holding capacity and nutrient density.

Example: Adding compost and aged manure to your garden bed before planting herbs like lavender and sage creates a nutrient-rich environment that promotes vigorous growth.

Soil Amendments

Amendments improve soil qualities to better fulfill the unique requirements of your herbs.

Improving Drainage

- Sand: Sand helps to enhance drainage and reduce waterlogging in thick clay soil. Add coarse sand to the top 6-8 inches of soil.
- perlite: Perlite, a lightweight volcanic rock, improves aeration and drainage. It's ideal for container gardening.

Example: If your garden soil is hard and compacted, add perlite or sand before planting rosemary and thyme, which appreciate well-drained soil.

Improving Nutrient Content

- Bone Meal: Bone meal is a slow-release source of phosphorus that is required for root development and blooming. Sprinkle bone meal in planting holes or incorporate it into the soil.
- Blood food: Blood food is a rapid source of nitrogen that promotes leafy development. Use it carefully to prevent overfertilization.
- Seaweed Extract Seaweed extract is high in trace nutrients and growth hormones, which improve plant health and resilience. Use it as a soil drench or

foliar spray.

Example: Using bone meal while planting herbs like chamomile and echinacea promotes robust root systems and profuse blossoms.

Balancing pH Levels

- Lime: To increase soil pH (making it more alkaline), add lime. This is beneficial for herbs that thrive in neutral to slightly alkaline environments.
- Sulfur: Add sulfur to lower the pH of the soil, making it more acidic. This helps to produce an ideal habitat for acid-loving herbs.

Example: If your soil test reveals acidic conditions, adding lime might help balance the pH for herbs like thyme and oregano, which prefer neutral to slightly alkaline soil.

Proper soil preparation and the correct amendments are essential for growing a flourishing herb garden. Understanding soil health, methodically preparing your garden beds or containers, and applying appropriate nutrients create an environment in which your medicinal herbs can thrive and produce potent, health-boosting substances

ORGANIC GARDENING PRACTICES.

Organic gardening is a comprehensive approach to plant cultivation that prioritizes sustainability, biodiversity, and environmental responsibility. Adopting organic practices in your herbal garden not only results in healthier, more potent herbs, but also benefits the ecosystem. This chapter looks at numerous organic growing strategies that will help your medicinal herbs thrive without the use of synthetic chemicals. We'll go over important methods that match with organic gardening concepts, including soil health and pest management.

Building Healthy Soil

The foundation of organic gardening is to cultivate good soil, which in turn fosters robust plant growth.

Composting

Composting is the recycling of organic matter into nutrient-dense humus, which improves soil fertility and structure.

- Materials: Combine kitchen wastes (fruit and vegetable peels, coffee grounds), yard debris (leaves, grass clippings), and other organic materials.
- Processing: Create a compost pile or bin by layering green (nitrogen-rich) and brown (carbon-

rich) materials. Keep the pile moist and turn it on a regular basis to promote aeration.
- Benefits: Compost enhances soil with nutrients, increases moisture retention, and promotes beneficial microbial activity.

Example: Adding homemade compost to your herb garden bed ensures a consistent source of nutrients for herbs such as basil and mint, fostering rapid growth.

Mulching.

Mulching is the process of covering the soil with organic materials to conserve moisture, control weeds, and promote soil health.

- Materials: Use straw, grass clippings, wood chips, or shredded leaves for mulch.
- Application: Place a 2-3 inch layer of mulch around your herbs to prevent direct contact with the stems.
- Benefits: Mulch helps keep soil hydrated, minimizes erosion, and adds organic matter as it decomposes.

Example: Mulching around lavender and rosemary plants helps maintain soil moisture levels, which is critical for these drought-tolerant herbs in hot areas.

Natural Fertilizers.

Organic fertilizers give critical nutrients to plants while avoiding the negative impacts of synthetic chemicals.

Manure.

Well-rotted animal dung is an excellent source of nutrients and organic materials.

- Types: Apply cow, horse, chicken, or sheep manure. To avoid burning plants, make sure it's properly composted.
- Application: Mix manure into the soil before planting or apply it as a top dressing during the growing season.
- Benefits: Manure enhances soil structure, fertility, and microbiological activity.

Example: Adding composted chicken manure to your herb garden promotes the growth of nutrient-dense herbs like parsley and cilantro.

Green manure

Green manure is the process of growing certain plants to increase soil fertility and structure.

- Plants: Use legumes (clover, alfalfa) and cover

crops (rye, buckwheat) for green manure.
- Process: Sow green manure plants in your garden bed, let them flourish, and then till them into the soil before planting herbs.
- Benefits: Green manure increases organic matter, fixes nitrogen, and improves soil texture.

Example: Planting clover as a green manure crop during the off-season increases soil nitrogen levels, which benefits heavy feeders like dill and fennel.

Organic Pest Management

Organic gardening stresses natural pest and disease management methods, hence fostering a healthy ecology.

Companion Planting

Companion planting entails growing particular plants together to promote growth and deter pests.

- Beneficial Pairings: Combining herbs and suitable plants can improve growth and pest resistance. For example, basil and tomatoes complement each other.
- Pest Deterrents: Certain plants naturally repel pests. Marigolds inhibit aphids and nematodes, whilst garlic repels a wide range of insects.
- Benefits: Companion planting decreases the demand for chemical pesticides while increasing

biodiversity.

Example: Planting basil near tomato plants repels tomato hornworms while also improving tomato quality.

Natural Predators

Encouraging natural predators helps keep insect populations under control without the use of chemicals.

- Beneficial Insects: Ladybugs, lacewings, and predatory beetles eat typical garden pests such as aphids and caterpillars.
- Habitat Creation: Planting flowers such as yarrow, dill, and fennel will attract beneficial insects to your garden.
- Benefits: Natural predators help to minimize pest numbers and maintain a balanced ecology.

Example: Introducing ladybugs to your herb garden can help decrease aphid infestations on plants such as parsley and chives.

Organic Sprays

Homemade sprays manufactured from natural substances can efficiently control pests and diseases.

- Insecticidal Soap: Combine water and a few drops of liquid soap to make a spray that kills soft-bodied insects such as aphids and mites.
- Neem Oil: Neem oil, obtained from the neem tree, serves as a natural pesticide and fungicide. Dilute and sprinkle it on the afflicted plants.
- Benefits: Organic sprays reduce harm to beneficial insects and the environment.

Example: Spraying neem oil on mint plants helps prevent spider mites without leaving any hazardous leftovers.

Water Conservation.

Efficient water utilization is an important part of sustainable organic agriculture.

Drip Irrigation

Drip irrigation directs water to the plant roots, reducing waste and evaporation.

- Installation: Set up a drip irrigation system using tubing and emitters to supply water slowly and accurately.
- Benefits: Drip irrigation saves water, reduces soil erosion, and lowers the risk of fungal disease.

Example: Drip irrigation in your herb garden

provides regular moisture to herbs like thyme and oregano, which love dry conditions.

Rainwater Harvesting

Collecting and using rainwater is an environmentally beneficial approach to water your plants.

- Systems: Use rain barrels or cisterns to collect runoff from your roof.
- Application: Use collected rainwater to irrigate your herbs, decreasing your reliance on municipal water sources.
- Benefits: Rainwater is chemical-free and perfect for plants, and harvesting lowers water bills while conserving natural resources.

Example: Watering your herb garden with rainwater offers a natural, chemical-free source of hydration for plants like lemon balm and chamomile.

Using organic gardening techniques in your herb garden encourages healthier plants, a more sustainable ecosystem, and a safer, chemical-free growing method. By cultivating good soil, employing natural fertilizers, organic pest management, and saving water, you may create a robust ecosystem in which your medicinal herbs can flourish. As you include these practices into your gardening routine, you'll reap the benefits of a healthy, productive, and ecologically friendly herb garden.

SELECTING MEDICAL HERBS TO GROW

Popular Medicinal Herbs for Beginners

Starting your own herbal garden may be an exciting and gratifying experience, especially if you select the correct therapeutic herbs to cultivate. As a beginner, it is critical to choose herbs that are easy to grow, hardy, and flexible in their applications. In this part, we'll look at some of the most popular and beginner-friendly therapeutic herbs. These herbs not only grow with minimal care, but they also provide a variety of health advantages that can be obtained directly from your garden.

Best Medicinal Herbs for Beginners

Basil (Ocimum Basilicum)

Basil is a fragrant herb that is widely used in culinary preparations, but it also has medicinal benefits.

- Growing Conditions: Prefers full sunlight and well-drained soil. Water regularly, especially during dry spells.
- Medicinal Applications: Known for its anti-inflammatory and antioxidant effects. Basil tea can

help with stress and digestion problems.
- Harvesting Tip: Pinching the leaves on a regular basis will encourage bushy growth. Harvest before flowering to maximize flavor and intensity.

Example: Prepare a calming tea with fresh basil leaves to help relieve headaches and anxiety.

Mint (mentha spp.)

Mint is a tough herb that spreads quickly and can be grown in pots to limit its size.

- Growing Conditions: Prefers moderate shade to full sun and wet, well-drained soil. Keep it controlled to avoid spreading.
- Medicinal Use: Mint is great for digestion, nausea, and sore throats. It can also be used in teas and inhalations to provide respiratory relief.
- Harvesting Tip: Trim the plant on a regular basis to keep it from becoming too long. For the finest flavor, harvest the leaves shortly before they blossom.

Example: Make a cup of mint tea to alleviate stomach, or steam fresh mint leaves to clear nasal congestion.

Chamomile (Matricaria Chamomilla)

Chamomile is a mild herb recognized for its calming properties.

- Growing Conditions: Prefers full sunlight and well-drained soil. Chamomile is drought-tolerant once established.
- Medicinal Use: Chamomile tea is commonly used for its relaxing properties, which can assist with insomnia, anxiety, and stomach difficulties. It also contains anti-inflammatory effects.
- Harvesting Tip: Harvest the blossoms when they are fully open and dry them for future use.

Example: A cup of chamomile tea before bed will help you relax and sleep better.

Lavender (Lavandula spp.)

Lavender is a gorgeous, aromatic herb that is both healthy and visually appealing.

- Growing Conditions: Needs full light and well-drained soil. Lavender is drought tolerant and prefers slightly alkaline soil.
- Medicinal Applications: Recognized for its soothing and antibacterial effects. Lavender oil can be used to treat stress, headaches, mild burns, and insect bites.
- Harvesting Tip: Harvest the flower spikes after they have fully bloomed. Dry them for use in

sachets, teas, or as an essential oil.

Example: Place dried lavender flowers in a sachet under your pillow to promote comfortable sleep, or add lavender oil to a bath to relax.

Lemon Balm (Melissa officinalis)

Lemon balm is a citrus-scented herb that is easy to grow and has numerous medical use.

- Growing Conditions: Prefers full sun to partial shade with wet, well-drained soil. It is hardy and can withstand a wide range of environments.
- Medicinal Use: Lemon balm is known for its soothing properties, which can help reduce anxiety, enhance sleep, and alleviate intestinal problems. It also contains antiviral properties.
- Harvesting Tip: Regularly pluck the leaves to keep the plant from growing too woody. The leaves can be utilized either fresh or dried.

Example: Lemon balm tea is a wonderful method to relax and relieve an upset stomach.

Echinacea (Echinacea Purpurea)

Echinacea, often called coneflower, is well-known for its immune-boosting effects.

- Growing Conditions: Prefers full sunlight and well-drained soil. It is drought tolerant and can withstand poor soil conditions.
- Medicinal Applications: Typically used to prevent and treat colds and flu. It stimulates the immune system, reduces inflammation, and is antiviral.
- Harvesting Tip: When the plant has reached maturity, harvest its blossoms and roots. Dry them to make teas, tinctures, or capsules.

Example: Make echinacea tea or tincture at the first sign of a cold to improve your immune system and lessen the intensity of symptoms.

Tips for Beginners

Start small.

To avoid getting overwhelmcd, start with a few easy-to-grow herbs.
- Concentrate on plants those you use frequently or want to learn more about for their therapeutic properties.

Example: Planting a tiny container garden with basil, mint, and chamomile is a practical way to begin your herbal gardening experience.

Learn and Experiment

- Familiarize yourself with each herb's growing requirements, therapeutic use, and harvesting methods.
- Experiment with various growth methods and recipes to see what works best for you and your garden.

Example: Try producing your own herbal teas, salves, and tinctures from the herbs you cultivate, and see how they affect your health.

Patience and consistency.

- Gardening demands patience and consistent attention. Regularly water, weed, and inspect your herbs for pests and diseases.
- Celebrate small victories and learn from any obstacles you face.

Example: Keep a gardening journal to follow the progress of your herbs, noting what works best and any changes you make along the way.

Starting your own medicinal herb garden can be a joyful and inspiring experience, especially if you choose beginner-friendly herbs such as basil, mint, chamomile, lavender, lemon balm, and echinacea. These herbs not only grow easily but also provide several health benefits. By starting small, learning as you go, and being patient, you may create a vibrant herb garden that improves your health and connects you with nature.

HERB PROFILES: USES AND BENEFITS

Understanding the distinct traits, uses, and benefits of medicinal herbs is essential when choosing the perfect ones for your garden. This chapter will provide thorough profiles of popular medicinal herbs, emphasizing their therapeutic powers, traditional uses, and practical applications. Understanding these herbs will allow you to make more informed decisions about which plants to grow and how to incorporate them into your daily wellness practice. Let's delve into the intriguing world of medicinal plants and uncover their potential to improve our health and well-being.

Herb Profiles.

Basil (Ocimum Basilicum)

Basil is a multipurpose herb prized for its fragrant leaves and therapeutic capabilities.

- Properties: Anti-inflammatory, antioxidant, antibacterial, and adaptogen.
- Uses: - Stress Relief: Basil tea or essential oil can help you feel less stressed and anxious.
- Digestive Health: Basil can help digestion and

relieve stomach pains.
- Support for the respiratory system: Basil has been used to cure colds, coughs, and respiratory illnesses.

Example: For a calming basil tea, soak fresh basil leaves in boiling water for 5-10 minutes. Drink to reduce tension and encourage relaxation.

Mint (mentha spp.)

Mint is a pleasant herb with a wide range of medical benefits.

- Properties: antispasmodic, carminative, and analgesic.
- Uses: - Digestive Aid: Mint tea can relieve indigestion, bloating, and gas.
- Pain Relief: Applying mint oil to the skin might help alleviate headaches and muscle pain.
- Respiratory Relief: Mint's menthol component helps to alleviate nasal congestion.

Example: Make a mint tea by steeping fresh or dried mint leaves in boiling water. This tea can assist to alleviate intestinal discomfort and refresh breath.

Chamomile (Matricaria Chamomilla)

Chamomile is a mild, calming herb that is commonly used to aid relaxation and sleep.

- Properties: antispasmodic, anti-inflammatory, and sedative.
- Uses: - Sleep Aid: Chamomile tea is well-known for enhancing sleep quality.
- Digestive Health: It can help relieve stomach discomfort and digestive problems.
- Skin Care: Chamomile-infused oils or creams can relieve skin irritations and eczema.

Example: Before bedtime, drink a cup of chamomile tea to relax and encourage restful sleep.

Lavender (Lavandula spp.)

Lavender is a fragrant herb known for its relaxing properties and versatility.

- Properties: antiseptic, anti-inflammatory, and sedative.
- Uses: - tension Relief: Lavender essential oil is widely used in aromatherapy to alleviate tension and anxiety.
- Skin Health: Applying lavender oil can help relieve burns, bug bites, and minor cuts.
- Sleep Aid: Lavender sachets or sprays can help improve sleep quality.

Example: Pour a few drops of lavender essential oil into your bath water for a soothing soak that relieves stress and anxiety.

Lemon Balm (Melissa officinalis)

Lemon balm is a citrus-scented herb with soothing and antiviral qualities.

- Properties: antiviral, antioxidant, and relaxing. Lemon balm tea or tincture can alleviate anxiety and promote tranquility.
- Digestive Health: It can help relieve indigestion and bloating.
- Cold sores: Applying lemon balm extract to cold sores helps hasten recovery.

Example: Prepare a lemon balm infusion by steeping fresh leaves in boiling water. Drink to reduce stress and improve your mood.

Echinacea (Echinacea Purpurea)

Echinacea is a potent immune-boosting herb used to prevent and treat illnesses.

- Properties: immunostimulant, anti-inflammatory, and antiviral.
- Uses: - Immune Support: Echinacea tea or tincture can strengthen the immune system and aid in the battle against colds and flu.
- Wound Healing: Echinacea poultices can be used

to cuts and wounds to aid in healing.
- Respiratory Health: It can help relieve symptoms
of respiratory infections.

Example: Drink echinacea tea as soon as you notice
symptoms of a cold to boost your immune system
and lessen the severity of the illness.

Practical Applications

Making Herbal Teas

Herbal teas are a simple and effective approach to
get the advantages of medicinal plants.

- Preparation: Choose fresh or dried herbs. Soak 1-2
teaspoons of dried herbs (or a handful of fresh
herbs) in boiling water for 5-10 minutes.
- Consumption: Consume 1-3 cups every day,
depending on the herb and your needs.

Example: A cup of chamomile tea before bedtime
can help you sleep better, and mint tea after dinner
can help you digest.

Making Herbal Tinctures

Tinctures are concentrated botanical extracts
prepared using alcohol or glycerin.

- preparation: Fill a container with chopped fresh or dried herbs. Cover with vodka, brandy, or glycerin. Seal and keep in a dark spot for 4-6 weeks, shaking daily.
- Utilization: Take 1-2 droppersful (about 30-60 drops) 2-3 times per day, diluted in water or juice.

Example: To increase immune function, use echinacea tincture when cold symptoms first appear.

Infusing Oils and Balms

Herbal oils and balms are applied topically to address skin ailments and pain.

- preparation: Fill a container with dried herbs and top with a carrier oil (such olive or coconut oil). Seal and store in a warm, sunny area for 2-3 weeks, shaking occasionally. Strain the infused oil and use it as is, or use it to balms and salves.
- Apply: Apply the infused oil or balm to the affected region two to three times daily.

Example: Lavender-infused oil can be used to soothe sunburns, while chamomile balm can help with eczema.

Understanding the uses and advantages of medicinal herbs allows you to make more informed decisions about which plants to produce and how to use them effectively. Making herbal teas, tinctures, or infused oils allows you to harness nature's healing power. By introducing these famous medicinal herbs into your garden and daily routine, you may improve your health and get the numerous therapeutic benefits they provide. Happy gardening and herbal healing!

SOURCING QUALITY SEEDS AND PLANTS.

Creating a therapeutic herb garden begins with getting high-quality seeds and plants. The quality of your original plant material has a tremendous impact on your garden's health, potency, and success. This chapter will walk you through the process of choosing and sourcing the best seeds and plants, guaranteeing a successful start to your herbal gardening experience. We will discuss where to buy, what to search for, and how to select the best solutions for your unique need.

Where To Buy

Local Nurseries and Garden Centers

Local nurseries and garden centers are fantastic places to buy quality plants and seeds.

- Benefits: - Expert guidance from local staff on growing conditions.

- The ability to examine plants in person for evidence of health and vitality.
- Supporting local businesses while lowering the environmental impact of shipping.

Example: Visit a nearby nursery to select healthy basil and mint plants that are free of pests and disease.

Online Retailers

Online shops sell a vast range of seeds and plants, including many uncommon or hard-to-find types.

- Benefits: - Wide range of therapeutic herbs from diverse places.
- Home delivery is convenient, and it generally comes with thorough planting and care instructions.
- Access to customer reviews and ratings to make informed purchasing selections.

Example: Purchase organic chamomile seeds from a reliable internet retailer specializing in medicinal herbs to ensure excellent germination rates and purity.

Seed Exchanges and Plant Swaps

Seed exchanges and plant swaps are community-organized activities in which gardeners exchange seeds and plants.

- Benefits: - Access to regionally tailored cultivars suitable for your climate.
- An inexpensive approach to diversity your garden.
- Making contacts with other gardeners and sharing information.

Example: Take part in a local seed swap to get heirloom echinacea seeds that are well-suited to your region's growing circumstances.

What to Look For

Seed Quality

Choosing high-quality seeds is essential for optimal germination and healthy plant growth.

- Factors to Consider: - Germination Rate: Select seeds with a high germination rate, which is usually noted on the seed packet.
- Organic Certification: Choose organic seeds free of synthetic chemicals and genetically modified organisms (GMOs).
- Freshness: Check the packaging date to ensure the seeds are fresh. Older seeds may have diminished viability.

Example: For best results, get fresh, organic

lavender seeds with a high germination rate from a reliable supplier.

Plant Health

When purchasing plants, carefully inspect them to ensure they are healthy and free of pests and illnesses.

- Indicators of Health: - Vigorous Growth: Observe strong stems, vivid leaves, and a well-developed root system.
- Pest-Free: Avoid plants that show apparent pests, webs, or evidence of harm.
- Disease-Free: Look for discoloration, spots, or wilting that could indicate disease.

Example: Choose a lemon balm plant with bright green leaves, no symptoms of yellowing, and a strong root system for transplantation into your garden.

How To Choose

Consider your climate and soil.

Herbs have different climate and soil requirements. Choose herbs that are appropriate for your local area.

- Climate Compatibility: Choose herbs appropriate for your hardiness zone and regular weather patterns.
- Soil Preferences: Make sure your soil type (e.g., sandy, loamy, clay) meets the requirements of the herbs you intend to plant.

Example: In a sunny, dry area, choose drought-tolerant herbs such as lavender and echinacea, which grow in well-drained soil.

Begin with easy-to-grow varieties.

Begin with herbs known for their tenacity and ease of cultivation.

- Beginner-Friendly Herbs: Basil, mint, and chamomile are great choices for beginner gardeners.
- Low Maintenance: Select herbs that need little attention and are resistant to common pests and diseases.

Example: Plant basil and mint in containers to manage their development and enjoy fresh herbs with little effort.

Seek Reliable Sources

Buy seeds and plants from reliable sellers to assure quality and authenticity.

- Reputable vendors: Purchase from well-known nurseries, garden centers, and online vendors with high ratings.
- Certified Seed: Look for certifications like organic, non-GMO, and heritage to ensure quality.

For example, order from a certified organic seed source that ensures non-GMO seeds for your therapeutic herb garden.

Practical Tips

Storing Seeds

Proper seed storage improves the survival and viability of subsequent plantings.

- Storage Conditions: Store seeds in a cool, dry place out of direct sunlight.
- Containers: Use airtight containers to avoid moisture and pest damage.

Example: To keep echinacea seeds dry and extend their shelf life, store them in a labeled glass jar with a silica gel packet.

Acclimatizing Plants

To prevent transplant shock, gradually introduce

new plants into your landscape.

- Hardening Off: Gradually expose plants to outdoor conditions throughout a week, beginning with a few hours of sunlight per day.
- Transplanting: Transplant on a cloudy day or in the evening to reduce stress from direct sunlight.

Example: Before transplanting your chamomile seedlings into your garden, acclimate them by exposing them to increasing amounts of sunlight every day.

Sourcing high-quality seeds and plants is an essential step in starting a healthy medicinal herb garden. By selecting the proper suppliers, selecting healthy and suitable types, and adhering to best storage and acclimation techniques, you may ensure a successful and happy gardening experience. Whether you get your herbs from local nurscrics, internet vendors, or community swaps, the time you spend into choosing quality ingredients will pay off in the shape of strong, productive plants that improve your health and well-being.

COMPANION PLANTING FOR HERBAL GARDENS

Companion planting is an ancient gardening strategy that combines diverse plants to promote growth, prevent pests, and improve overall garden health. Companion planting is very advantageous in herbal gardens because it promotes biodiversity, maximizes space, and creates a harmonious growing environment. This chapter will look at the fundamentals of companion planting, highlight advantageous herb pairings, and offer practical advice for successfully adopting this method in your herbal garden.

The advantages of companion planting

Pest Control

Certain plants have natural insect repellent properties, which protect your therapeutic herbs from damage.

- Natural Deterrents: Certain herbs produce smells that confuse or repel pests, decreasing the need for chemical pesticides.
- The Predator Attraction: Companion plants can attract helpful insects like ladybugs and lacewings, which eat pests.

Example: Marigolds, with their strong aroma, can repel aphids and nematodes from your herbs.

Enhanced Growth and Flavor

Companion planting can improve the growth and quality of your herbs.

- Nutrient Sharing: Some plants improve soil nutrients, hence benefiting surrounding plants via nutrient uptake.
- Microclimate Creation: Taller plants can provide shade for sensitive herbs, resulting in a pleasant microclimate.

Example: Basil pairs nicely with tomatoes since it not only improves the flavor of the tomatoes but also benefits from the shade offered by larger plants.

Biodiversity and Resilience

Growing a diverse set of plants fosters a healthy and resilient garden environment.

- Soil Health: Diverse plant roots enhance soil structure and fertility, resulting in healthier plants.
- Disease Prevention: A diversified garden can help slow the development of illnesses and pests that thrive in monocultures.

Example: A garden with a variety of herbs, flowers, and vegetables may produce a balanced ecology that promotes healthy growth.

Companion Planting Strategies

Selecting Compatible Herbs

Selecting the appropriate herb combinations is critical for successful companion planting.

- comparable Growing Requirements: For best results, pair herbs that require comparable amounts of water and light.
- Complementary Growth Habits: Combine plants that complement one another, such as taller plants providing shade for lower-growing herbs.

Example: Chamomile attracts helpful insects and aids in the growth of broccoli, making it a good combination.

Incorporating Flowers and Vegetables

Flowers and veggies can enhance your herbal garden by attracting beneficial insects and pollinators.

- Companion Flowers: Plant flowers such as calendula, nasturtium, and borage beside your herbs to attract pollinators and repel pests.
- Vegetable Companion: Many vegetables complement herbs well, providing mutual benefits in pest control and nutrition exchange.

Example: Planting nasturtiums beside your herbs

attracts pollinators while also repelling aphids and other common pests.

Companion Planting Pairings

1. Basil and tomatoes.

- Benefits: Basil improves the flavor of tomatoes and repels pests such as aphids and whiteflies.
- Growing Tip: Plant basil near tomatoes to benefit from their complementing growth patterns.

2: Chamomile with Cabbage

- Benefits: Chamomile attracts helpful insects and promotes cabbage growth.
- Growing Tip: Spread chamomile seeds around your cabbage plants to form a healthy connection.

3: Mint and Cabbage Family

- Benefits: Mint repels cabbage moths and other cabbage-related pests.
- Growing Tip: Plant mint along the perimeter of your cabbage patch to provide natural crop protection.

4. Lavender with Rosemary

- Benefits: Lavender and rosemary attract pollinators

and repel pests, making them ideal companions.
- Growing Tip: Plant them together in sunny areas
for a fragrant and healthful combo.

Practical Tips for Companion Planting.

Plan Your Layout

- Garden Design: Plan out your garden layout,
noting where you will plant various herbs, flowers,
and vegetables to reap the most benefits of
companion planting.
- Spacing: Make sure that plants have enough room
to grow without overcrowding, which can lead to
resource competition.

Example: Create a companion planting chart to see
how your herbs, flowers, and veggies will be
organized.

Monitor and adjust.

- Observation: Check your garden on a regular basis
for symptoms of pests or poor growth. Adjust your
companion plantings as necessary.
- Rotation: Rotate your herb buddies every season to
reduce pest and disease development.

Example: If you find a pest problem with one herb,
try swapping it out for the next growing season to

boost plant health.

Companion planting is an effective approach for improving the health and productivity of your herb garden. By choosing appropriate herbs, including beneficial flowers and vegetables, and carefully arranging your garden layout, you can create a vibrant ecosystem that encourages growth, repels pests, and nurtures resilience. Adopt the practice of companion planting and watch your medicinal herbs thrive alongside their helpful companions, enriching both your garden and your wellness journey

PLANTING AND GROWING MEDICAL HERBS

Starting Herbs from Seed

Starting your medicinal herbs from seeds is an exciting and fulfilling adventure that allows you to reconnect with nature while also nurturing your garden from the ground up. This chapter will walk you through the process of planting seeds, ensuring that you have the information and equipment needed for effective germination and growth. From choosing the correct seeds to understanding planting techniques and care, we'll cover everything you need to start your herbal garden growing.

Choosing the Right Seeds.

Selecting Quality Seeds.

The quality of the seeds you use will determine the success of your herb garden.

- Source from reputable suppliers: Choose seeds from reputable nurseries or internet vendors known for their quality and purity.
- Check for Certification: Organic and non-GMO certifications guarantee that you're sowing healthy, chemical-free seeds.
- Read the reviews: Customer evaluations might

provide information about germination rates and general satisfaction.

Example: Buy organic basil seeds from a respected seed source to ensure high germination and disease resistance.

Understanding Seed Varieties

Herbs are classified into many different types, each with its own set of traits and growth patterns.

- Heirloom vs. Hybrid: Heirloom seeds are open-pollinated and have been passed down through generations, whereas hybrids may provide specific qualities but do not produce true-to-type offspring.
- Choose Varieties Suitable for Your Climate: Choose herbs that flourish in your local growing conditions, taking into account aspects such as hardiness zone, sunlight, and moisture content.

Example: If you reside in a warm region, try planting heat-tolerant herbs such as oregano and thyme.

Preparing to Plant

Gather your supplies.

Before planting, gather all of the supplies you'll

need to create the best environment for your seeds.

- Containers: Plant your seeds in seed trays, pots, or recycled containers with drainage holes.
- Seed Starting Mix: A lightweight, sterile seed starting mix creates an optimal atmosphere for germination.
- Labelling: Keep track of your seeds by identifying them with the herb's name and sowing date.

Example: Use egg cartons as seedling trays, ensuring that each compartment includes drainage holes.

Determine the Planting Time

For successful germination and growth, seed sowing must be timed correctly.

- Check Seed Packets: Most seed packets include instructions on the optimal planting period, such as when to start indoors and when to transplant outside.
- Consider Your Final Frost Date: For outdoor planting, begin seeds indoors 6-8 weeks before the latest frost date in your location.

Example: If your final frost date is April 15, plant basil seeds indoors in early March for the best growth season.

Planting Seeds

Sowing Techniques

Once your seeds and supplies are ready, it's time to plant them.

- Planting Depth: Refer to the seed packet directions for the proper planting depth, as each herb has its own requirements.
- Spacing: Leave enough spacing between seeds to avoid overcrowding and promote good air circulation.
- Watering: After planting, lightly sprinkle the soil to keep it evenly moist without overwatering.

Example: Sow chamomile seeds about 1/4 inch deep and 12 inches apart to allow for its development habit.

Germination Environment

Creating the ideal atmosphere for germination is critical to effective seed beginning.

- temperature: Most seeds germinate best in temperatures ranging from 65°F to 75°F (18°C to 24°C). Use a heat mat if necessary.
- LIGHT: Once the seeds have germinated, provide enough of light, either from natural sunlight or grow

lights, for 12-16 hours per day.
- HUMIDITY: Covering containers with plastic wrap or a humidity dome can help keep moisture in until the seeds germinate.

Example: To ensure optimal germination conditions, place your seed trays on a warm windowsill or beneath grow lights.

Care for Seedlings

Watering and Feeding

Proper care is required as your seedlings grow to ensure their healthy development.

- Watering: Keep the soil regularly moist but not overly wet. Water gradually to avoid disrupting the seeds.
- Fertilization: After a few weeks, begin feeding seedlings with a diluted liquid fertilizer to encourage healthy growth.

Example: Every 2-4 weeks, use a balanced organic fertilizer to guarantee your seedlings obtain critical nutrients.

Thinning Seedlings

To avoid overpopulation, trim seedlings once they

produce their first true leaves.

- Select the Strongest Seedlings: Snip weaker seedlings at the root with scissors, allowing only the healthiest to thrive.
- Space Appropriately: Follow the recommended spacing for each herb to ensure they have enough area to grow.

Example: If you sowed numerous basil seeds in a single pot, trim them down to one or two strong plants to ensure robust growth.

Transplant Seedlings

Timing for Transplantation

When your seedlings have formed strong roots and are about 2-4 inches tall, they are ready to be transplanted outside.

- Hardening Off: Gradually adapt seedlings to outdoor circumstances over a week, beginning with a few hours of sunlight per day.
- Soil Preparation: Fill your garden bed or containers with well-drained soil rich in organic matter.

Example: Begin hardening off your chamomile seedlings a week before the latest frost date by putting them outside for longer periods of time each day.

Transplantation Technique

When transplanting, follow these procedures to success:

- Dig Holes: Make holes in the garden bed or container that are somewhat larger than each seedling's root ball.
- Remove Carefully: Gently remove seedlings from their containers, taking care not to injure the roots.
- Plant at the Same Depth: Place seedlings in holes at the same depth as they were in their pots, then backfill with dirt and thoroughly water.

Example: When transplanting mint, keep the soil moist to help the roots settle in their new surroundings.

Starting herbs from seeds is a gratifying experience that allows you to produce your own therapeutic plants from the start. By choosing quality seeds, preparing for planting, and giving adequate care, you may lay the groundwork for a healthy herbal garden. Accept the joy of caring for your plants and watch them grow from small seeds to sturdy, healthy herbs ready to help your wellness journey

TRANSPLANTING SEEDLINGS

Transplanting seedlings is an important stage in cultivating medicinal herbs because it allows young plants to thrive in their final developing environment. This approach can have a substantial impact on their health and productivity. Proper transplanting techniques guarantee that seedlings experience little shock and can grow robust roots in their new habitat. In this chapter, we'll go over the methods and best practices for transplanting seedlings, so you can effectively transition your young herbs from inside or the seed tray to the garden bed or larger pots.

Timing of Transplant

Determining the Right Time

Timing is critical for effective transplantation since it influences the seedlings' ability to adapt and thrive.

- Seedling Size: Transplant when seedlings reach 2-4 inches tall and have a strong set of true leaves.
- Weather Conditions: Select a gloomy day or transplant in the late afternoon to reduce stress from heat and sunlight.
- Last Frost Date: Confirm that the risk of frost has passed, particularly for fragile herbs.

Example: If you started basil seeds indoors and they are 3 inches tall with healthy leaves, wait until after the last frost to put them outside.

Preparing for Transplant

Hardening off

Hardening off is the slow acclimatization of seedlings to outdoor circumstances, which aids in their adaptation and decreases transplant shock.

- Process Duration: Begin hardening off 7-10 days before transplantation.
- Gradual Exposure: Begin by putting seedlings outside for a few hours each day, gradually increasing the time and exposure to sunlight.
- Sheltered Locations: Protect seedlings from high winds and direct sunlight for the first few days.

Example: Begin by putting your chamomile seedlings in a shady area outside for a few hours, then gradually exposing them to more sunlight each day.

Soil Preparation

Preparing the soil at the transplanting area is critical for providing the nutrients and environment that seedlings require to thrive.

- Soil Quality: Improve fertility and drainage by amending well-drained, nutrient-rich soil with organic matter such as compost.
- Tilling: Loosen the soil in the planting area to a depth of 12 inches to allow roots to penetrate readily.
- Moisture: Water the area a day or two before transplanting to maintain a wet but not soggy condition.

Example: Add compost to the garden plot where you intend to transplant basil to improve soil quality and nutritional content.

Transplantation Techniques

Tools and Supplies

To ensure a smooth and fast transplanting process, gather all necessary equipment and supplies before beginning.

- Tools: Use a trowel, transplanting fork, or hand spade to dig holes and relocate seedlings.
- Containers: Prepare pots or trays for any seedlings that need to be temporarily stored during the transplanting process.
- Watering Can: Fill a watering can with water for

quick hydration after transplanting.

Example: A little hand spade is ideal for digging holes for your mint seedlings while causing minimal disruption to their roots.

The Transplantation Process

Follow these steps to ensure a successful transplant:

1. Prepare the Holes: Dig holes twice as wide and as deep as each seedling's root ball. Space them according to the herb's specified distance.
2. Remove Seedlings: Gently remove seedlings from their containers or trays, being careful not to injure the roots. If they are root-bound, gently separate the roots to promote growth.
3. Place in Holes: Place the seedlings in the holes, making sure they are the same depth they were growing in their original containers.
4. Backfill and Firm: Fill the holes with soil, gently pressing down to eliminate air pockets and maintain proper soil contact with the roots.
5. Water Thoroughly: Water newly transplanted plants right away to help settle the soil and reduce transplant shock.

Example: When transplanting rosemary, make sure the roots are not twisted and set the seedling at the same soil level as it was in the container.

Post-transplant Care

Water and Mulching

Proper post-transplant care is crucial for seedlings to establish themselves in their new habitat.

- Watering: Keep the soil moist but not saturated for the first two weeks after transplanting.
- Mulching: Place a layer of organic mulch around the seedlings' base to help retain moisture and prevent weeds.

Example: Apply straw or shredded leaves as mulch around newly transplanted echinacea to keep the soil moist and preserve the young roots.

Monitoring Growth

Regularly check your transplanted seedlings for symptoms of stress, pests, or disease.

- Signs of Stress: Look for drooping, yellowing leaves, or stunted growth, which could suggest transplant shock or other problems.
- Pest Management: Check for pests and diseases and take the necessary precautions to safeguard your herbs.

Example: If you find your mint plants drooping after transplanting, make sure they're getting enough water and look for any root damage.

Transplanting seedlings is an important step in producing healthy medicinal plants. You may set your seedlings up for success by transplanting at the right time, preparing the soil, and using proper practices. With proper care and monitoring, your transplanted herbs will thrive in their new surroundings, ready to supply you with the natural benefits they offer. Embrace this gratifying process and watch your garden thrive as your therapeutic herbs grow vibrantly.

WATERING AND FERTILIZING HERBS

Watering and fertilizing are crucial for cultivating healthy medicinal herbs. Proper hydration and nutrition have a direct impact on plant growth, vigor, and yield. Understanding your herbs' specific watering and fertilizing requirements will help you cultivate a thriving garden full of aromatic and helpful plants. This chapter will go over recommended methods for watering and fertilizing your herbs, ensuring they get the care they need to thrive.

Watering Herbs

Understanding Water Needs

Herbs have different water requirements depending on their growth stage, climate, and soil conditions.

- Established vs. Newly Planted: Newly planted herbs typically require more regular watering until their roots develop, whilst older plants may demand less.
- Soil Type: Sandy soils drain fast and may require more frequent watering, whereas clay soils retain moisture for longer.
- Climate Conditions: Hot, dry weather causes evaporation, requiring more frequent watering.

Example: In warmer weather, basil, which needs continuously moist soil, may require daily watering, whereas rosemary, a drought-tolerant plant, may require only occasional watering.

Watering Techniques

Using the proper watering strategies will increase the health of your herbs while reducing water wastage.

- Deep Watering: Water deeply and infrequently to promote deep root growth. Aim for around 1 inch of water every week, whether from rain or irrigation.
- Soaker Hose and Drip Irrigation: These

technologies deliver water straight to the soil, reducing evaporation and ensuring moisture reaches the roots.
- Watering at the Appropriate Time: Water early in the morning or late in the afternoon to limit evaporation and avoid leaf scorch.

Example: Use a soaker hose in your herb garden to provide continuous moisture directly to the roots, particularly during the hot summer months.

Signs of Overwatering and Underwatering

Recognizing the indicators of water stress might help you modify your watering habits quickly.

- Overwatering Symptoms: Yellowing leaves, withering in damp soil, and root rot are all indicators of too much moisture.
- Underwatering Symptoms: Wilting leaves, dry soil, and browning leaf tips suggest that your herbs require additional water.

Example: If your cilantro is withering and the soil seems moist, you should reduce watering to avoid root rot.

Fertilizing Herbs

Understanding Nutritional Needs

Herbs often require fewer nutrients than other garden plants, but a well-balanced fertilizer can boost growth and flavor.

- Soil Testing: Perform a soil test to evaluate nutrient levels and pH, which will help you to adjust your fertilization strategy.
- N-P-K Ratios: Select fertilizers with balanced N-P-K (nitrogen, phosphorus, and potassium) ratios to encourage healthy leaf and root development.

Example: Most herbs benefit from a balanced fertilizer with an N-P-K ratio of 10-10-10, which promotes vigorous growth while avoiding excessive leafiness.

Types of Fertilizers

Choose the appropriate fertilizer based on your herbs' demands and growing philosophy.

- Organic Options: Compost, well-rotted manure, fish emulsion, and seaweed extract all add nutrients while boosting soil health.
- Synthetic Options: Chemical fertilizers provide immediate nutrient availability but may not improve soil structure or health over time.

Example: Using compost tea as a natural fertilizer in

your herb garden can increase nutrient levels and soil microbial activity.

Fertilizing Techniques

Applying fertilizer appropriately is critical for optimizing its advantages and avoiding plant stress.

- Timing: Fertilize at the start of the growing season and again in mid-summer, especially for herbs that grow quickly, such as basil and cilantro.
- Application method: Granular fertilizers should be used as directed on the container, either mixed into the soil or as a top dressing. Liquid fertilizers should be diluted to half strength and applied with regular watering.

Example: To fertilize thyme, sprinkle a balanced organic fertilizer around the plant's base and lightly work it into the soil.

Signs of Nutrient Deficiency

Recognizing the symptoms of vitamin deficiency might help you address issues sooner.

- Nitrogen Deficiency: Yellowing leaves, particularly older ones, and slowed growth indicate a nitrogen shortage.
- Phosphorus Deficiency: Dark green or purplish

leaves and poor blossoming indicate a lack of phosphorus.
- Potassium shortage: Browning leaf edges and weakened stems are signs of a potassium shortage.

Example: If your oregano has yellowing leaves and reduced development, it may require nitrogen-rich fertilizer to recover.

Watering and fertilizing are essential activities for cultivating healthy medicinal herbs. Understanding your herbs' water requirements, using proper watering strategies, and providing appropriate nutrients can allow you to grow a vibrant garden full of aromatic and helpful plants. With proper hydration and nutrition, your medicinal herbs will thrive, providing you with the natural health benefits they are known for

MANAGING PESTS AND DISEASES

Managing pests and illnesses is an important component of growing quality medicinal herbs. While herbs can be tough and have natural defenses, they are nonetheless vulnerable to a variety of pests and illnesses that can harm their development and quality. Proactive management tactics not only safeguard your plants, but they also improve the general health of your garden environment. This chapter will go over practical ways for identifying, preventing, and treating pests and illnesses, so that your medicinal herbs can grow in a healthy and vibrant environment.

Understanding Common Pests

Identifying Common Herbal Pests

Early detection of pest infestations can help to avoid larger difficulties in the future. Here are some typical pests affecting therapeutic herbs:

Aphids are little, soft-bodied insects that swarm on new growth and suck sap, causing yellowing leaves.
- Spider Mites: These tiny, spider-like organisms produce fine webbing on plants and inflict stippled leaf damage.
- Whiteflies: These small, white flying insects feed on plant sap, causing weaker plants and sticky residue on leaves.
- Slugs and Snails: Soft-bodied pests that consume leaves, frequently leaving irregular holes and slime trails.

Example: If you detect wilting leaves on your basil plants, look for aphids hiding on the undersides.

Prevention of Pest Infestations

Developing a Healthy Garden Environment

Pest management relies heavily on prevention. Healthy growing habits can help prevent pests from invading your medicinal plants.

- Diversity: To enhance biodiversity, plant a range of herbs and companion plants, making pests less likely to thrive.
- Healthy Soil: Use well-drained, nutrient-rich soil to promote strong plant development and increase natural insect resistance.
- Regular monitoring: To detect pests or illness early on, inspect your plants on a regular basis.

Example: Incorporate flowering plants, such as marigolds, into your herb garden to attract beneficial insects like ladybugs and lacewings, which prey on pests.

Managing Pests

Organic Control Methods

If you have a pest problem, there are several organic ways to control it properly.

- Handpicking: For larger pests such as slugs and snails, handpicking is a simple and effective control technique.
- Insecticidal Soap: Use insecticidal soap or neem

oil to treat soft-bodied insects such as aphids and whitefly.
- Diatomaceous Earth: Sprinkle food-grade diatomaceous earth around your plants to provide a barrier that discourages crawling pests.

Example: To limit the amount of aphids without harming beneficial insects, apply neem oil to your cilantro plants as soon as they appear.

Identifying and Managing Diseases

Identifying Common Plant Diseases

Diseases, like pests, can pose a hazard to your herbs' health. The ability to detect common diseases is critical for effective management.

- Powdery Mildew: A white, powdery fungal growth on leaves that causes stunted growth and lower yields.
- Root Rot is caused by overwatering and poor drainage, resulting in wilted plants and blackened roots.
- Botrytis Blight (Gray Mold) is a fungal disease that causes gray mold to form on leaves, particularly under humid environments.

Example: If your oregano leaves are covered in white powder, they may have powdery mildew, which needs to be treated right once to prevent it from spreading.

Preventing Diseases

Best Practices for Disease Prevention

Implementing excellent cultural practices can dramatically lower the risk of disease in your herb crop.

- Proper Watering: Avoid overhead watering to reduce humidity and keep foliage dry, so preventing fungal diseases.
- Adequate space: Maintain adequate space between plants to encourage air circulation and reduce humidity levels.
- Cleanliness: Immediately remove any dead or diseased plant material to prevent pathogen transmission.

Example: Water your chamomile plants at the base rather than the top to reduce moisture on the leaves and prevent powdery mildew.

Managing Disease

Organic Treatments for Disease

If problems develop, there are organic therapy

alternatives available to assist restore the health of your herbs.

- Fungicides: Treat fungal infections with organic fungicides that contain substances such as potassium bicarbonate or sulfur.
- Homemade Remedies: Make a baking soda spray (1 teaspoon baking soda combined with 1 quart water) to treat powdery mildew.
- Crop Rotation: Crop rotation helps to prevent soil-borne diseases from recurring in the garden.

Example: To help reduce the spread of powdery mildew, spray your thyme plants with a baking soda solution as soon as the first signs appear.

Pest and disease control is critical to the success of your therapeutic herb garden. You can safeguard and ensure the health of your plants by remaining watchful and using prevention techniques. Whether you have pests or illnesses, there are a number of organic control methods available to assist you restore the health of your herbs. With a proactive approach and attention to detail, you may create a thriving garden full with aromatic and helpful plants

MAINTAINING YOUR HERB GARDEN

Pruning and Harvesting Techniques

A thriving herb garden demands consistent attention, especially when it comes to pruning and harvesting. These crucial techniques not only promote growth, but also improve the flavor and freshness of your herbs. Pruning shapes plants, removes dead or damaged foliage, and increases air circulation, whilst correct harvesting guarantees that your plants produce the most during the growth season. In this chapter, we'll look at how to prune and harvest effectively, giving you the knowledge and confidence you need to keep your herb garden healthy and prolific.

Pruning Techniques

Why prune?

Pruning is critical to the health and output of your herbs. Here's why this matters:

- Encourages Growth: Regular trimming promotes bushier growth and keeps plants from becoming lanky or overgrown.
- Removes Dead Material: Removing dead or diseased leaves helps to avoid the spread of illnesses and pests.

- Increases Air Circulation: Proper trimming improves airflow around the plant, lowering humidity and the danger of fungal disease.

Example: Pruning your basil on a regular basis will result in larger, more productive plants with more harvestable leaves.

When to prune

Knowing when to prune is critical for keeping your herbs healthy and productive.

- Spring: Pruning perennial plants like mint and oregano in the early spring promotes new growth.
- Before flowering: Prune annual herbs like basil and cilantro before they flower to keep their flavor and prevent them from going to seed.
- Throughout the Season: Check your herbs frequently and prune as needed to remove any dead or damaged leaves.

Example: In early spring, prune your rosemary by cutting back around one-third of the plant to promote new growth and maintain shape.

Pruning Techniques

Here are some efficient pruning techniques to implement in your herb garden.

- Pinching: Using your fingers, pinch off the top growth of soft-stemmed herbs such as basil and mint. This approach promotes bushier growth while preventing flowering.
- Cut: To cleanly cut woody herbs such as rosemary and thyme, use sharp, clean scissors or pruning shears. Cut right above a leaf node to stimulate new growth.
- Thinning: Remove any congested stems and leaves to enhance air circulation and allow sunlight to reach all areas of the plant.

Example: When pruning thyme, use scissors to cut stems slightly above a leaf node to encourage healthy branching and a fuller plant.

Harvesting Techniques

When to Harvest

Knowing when to harvest your herbs ensures the highest flavor and potency.

- Before Flowering: For the finest flavor, harvest herbs such as basil, dill, and cilantro right before they flower.
- Morning Harvest: The greatest time to harvest is in the morning, after the dew has dried but before the sun becomes too hot, because essential oils are at

their peak.

Example: Pick your mint in the morning for the most aromatic and tasty leaves.

Harvesting Techniques

Proper harvesting practices can extend the life of your herbs and provide the best flavor.

- Cutting Stems: Use sharp scissors to cut stems while being careful not to injure the plant. Always leave enough foliage to promote future growth.
- Harvesting Leaves: For leaf herbs such as parsley and cilantro, remove the outer leaves first, allowing the inner leaves to grow.
- Remove Flower: If your herbs start to flower, remove them to divert the plant's energy back to leaf formation.

Example: When picking cilantro, remove the outer leaves at the base of the stalk to allow the interior leaves to grow and continue producing.

How to Store and Use Fresh Herbs

Once your herbs have been collected, knowing how to store and use them correctly will improve your cooking experience.

- Fresh Use: To get the most flavor out of your herbs, use them right away. Chop or tear them immediately before adding to a dish.
- Drying: Drying herbs upside down in a cold, dark room or using a dehydrator can extend their shelf life. Store dried herbs in sealed containers away from direct sunlight.
- Freeze: Wash and chop the herbs, then freeze them in ice cube trays with a little water or olive oil. Once frozen, transfer to bags for convenient usage in soups and stews.

Example: To preserve fresh basil, cut the leaves and combine with olive oil before freezing in ice cube trays for later use in sauces and salads.

Pruning and harvesting are essential strategies for keeping a thriving herb garden. Understanding when and how to prune your herbs, as well as proper harvesting practices, will help to keep your plants healthy, productive, and flavorful. Regular adherence to these procedures not only improves the growth and quality of your herbs, but also increases the flavor of your culinary creations. Enjoy the process of caring for your herb garden, and reap the benefits of your labor

SEASONAL CARE AND MAINTENANCE.

Seasonal care and upkeep are essential for keeping

your herb garden healthy year-round. Each season presents unique difficulties and opportunities for your herbs' health and productivity. Understanding your plants' particular demands throughout the year allows you to give proper care and establish an atmosphere that promotes robust development. In this chapter, we'll look at seasonal herb garden maintenance strategies to keep your plants healthy and productive throughout the year.

Spring Care

Planning for New Growth

Spring is the season of regeneration and development in the garden. As temperatures rise, herbs awaken from their winter hibernation.

- Soil Preparation: Test your soil and add organic materials, such as compost, to boost fertility and drainage.
- Transplanting: If you started your seeds indoors, now is the moment to harden them by progressively exposing them to outdoor conditions before transplanting.
- Pruning: Remove dead or damaged foliage from perennial herbs to encourage healthy new growth.

Example: Pruning back any dead stems and modifying the soil with compost may help your thyme plants grow faster.

Planting New Herbs

Spring is the best season to add fresh herbs into your garden.

- Direct Seeding: After the latest frost date, sow seeds of annual herbs such as basil, cilantro, and dill straight into the soil.
- Choosing Varieties: Planting a range of herbs will offer a diverse crop throughout the season.

Example: Planting basil and cilantro together can add fresh flavors to your summer dishes while also increasing the output of your herb garden.

Summer Care.

Maintaining Growth

As the weather heats, your herbs will require regular attention to grow.

- Watering: Make sure to water your herbs on a regular basis, especially during hot, dry weather. Aim for about an inch of water every week, adjusted for rainfall.
- Mulching: Spread a layer of organic mulch to retain moisture, reduce weeds, and regulate soil

temperature.
- Pest Management: Keep an eye out for pests and diseases, and take proactive steps to address any issues that occur.

Example: During a heatwave, consider placing mulch around your basil plants to keep the soil cool and moisture levels stable.

Harvesting

Summer is the season of profuse growth, which makes it ideal for harvesting.

- Regular Harvesting: In annual herbs, harvest leaves and stems on a regular basis to promote bushier growth and prevent blossoming.
- Timing: Harvest in the morning when the essential oils are at their peak concentration for the finest flavor.

Example: Snip the tops of your mint plants on a regular basis to stimulate fuller development, while enjoying fresh mint in beverages and foods.

Fall Care

Preparing for Dormancy

As the weather cools, it's time to prepare your herb

garden for the winter.

- Final Harvest: Gather any remaining herbs before the first frost, as cold weather can harm leaves and reduce flavor.
- Cutting Back: To promote healthy regrowth in spring, trim back perennial herbs such as chives and oregano.
- Mulching for Protection: To protect perennial herbs' roots from cold weather, apply a layer of mulch.

Example: Before the first frost, harvest your remaining rosemary and thyme for drying or freezing to preserve their flavor for winter cooking.

Winter Care

Protecting Your Herbs

Winter can be a difficult season for your herb garden, particularly in colder locations.

- Indoor Transition: Move potted herbs indoors to protect plants from frost and lengthen their harvest.
- Covering Outdoor plants: Use row covers or frost blankets to protect hardy plants like parsley and sage from the cold.
- Monitoring Watering: If your herbs are kept inside, keep an eye on their moisture levels because the air

inside can be dryer.

Example: If you have potted basil and parsley, set them on a sunny ledge indoors to enjoy fresh herbs throughout winter.

Seasonal care and upkeep are essential for the health and productivity of your herb garden. By tailoring your gardening habits to the specific needs of each season, you can ensure that your herbs thrive and continue to produce flavorful and healthy foliage year-round. Embrace the changes that each season brings and reap the benefits of a well-kept herbal garden.

Mulching and Weed Control

Maintaining a healthy herb garden entails more than just planting and watering; efficient mulching and weed control are crucial for encouraging healthy growth. Mulching not only helps to maintain soil moisture and control temperature, but it also reduces weed development, giving your herbs the best conditions to thrive. On the other side, weed control is critical for ensuring that your herbs have access to the nutrients and minerals they require. In this chapter, we will look at the benefits of mulching, effective weed control tactics, and best practices for keeping your herb garden healthy.

The Benefits of Mulching

Why Use Mulch?

Mulching is one of the most effective ways to boost the health and productivity of your herb garden. Here are several significant advantages:

- Moisture Retention: Mulch helps keep soil moisture by minimizing evaporation, which is especially useful during the hot summer months.
- Temperature Regulation: A layer of mulch insulates the soil, making it colder in the summer and warmer in the winter, creating a stable climate for your herbs.
- Weed Suppression: Mulch blocks sunlight, preventing weed seeds from developing and considerably lowering the requirement for hand weeding.
- Soil Improvement: Organic mulches decompose over time, introducing nutrients and improving soil structure.

Example: A layer of straw mulch around your basil plants can help keep moisture levels stable, resulting in healthy growth throughout the summer.

Types of Mulch

Choosing the appropriate type of mulch is critical

for reaping its full advantages. Here are a few popular choices:

- Organic Mulches: Materials such as straw, shredded leaves, wood chips, and grass clippings degrade to improve soil quality.
- Inorganic Mulches: Materials such as plastic sheeting or landscaping cloth can efficiently reduce weeds while providing no nutrients to the soil.
- Living Mulches: Certain low-growing plants, such as clover, can operate as living mulch by suppressing weeds and providing ground cover.

Example: Using shredded leaves as mulch not only inhibits weeds but also enriches the soil as they decompose.

Effective Weed Control

Understanding Weeds

Weeds compete with your herbs for light, moisture, and nutrition. Recognizing typical weed types will allow you to efficiently manage them:

- Annual weeds: These weeds (such as crabgrass) finish their life cycle within a year. They can be controlled with careful weeding and mulching.
- Perennial weeds: These weeds (such as dandelions) return year after year. They necessitate more

persistent control efforts, including deep-root removal.

Example: Identifying dandelions in your herb garden is critical for proper management since they can spread rapidly and outcompete your herbs.

Manual Weeding Techniques

While mulching helps to control weeds, they will eventually appear. Here are several excellent hand weeding approaches.

- Hand Weeding: Check your herb garden on a regular basis and eradicate weeds by hand, making sure to pull them by the roots to avoid regrowth.
- Hoeing: Use a hoe to cut weeds at the soil's surface, inhibiting their growth while protecting your herbs.
- Mulching After Weeding: Spread a layer of mulch immediately after weeding to prevent new weeds from growing.

Example: Hand-weeding around your mint plants can help guarantee they have access to nutrients without being competed by weeds.

Tips for Mulching and Weed Control

When to Mulch

- Timing: Apply mulch in the spring after the soil has warmed but before the summer heat arrives. A 2-4 inch covering of mulch is recommended.
- Renewing Mulch: Every season, refresh your mulch layer, adding more as needed to keep it thick and effective.

Weeding regularly

- Consistency: Make weeding a regular component of your gardening schedule. Weed at least once a week to keep weeds under control.
- After Rain: Weeds are simpler to pull when the earth is damp, so take advantage of the natural watering.

Example: Schedule a weekly garden inspection on Sunday mornings to remain on top of any sprouting weeds.

Mulching and weed control are critical components of keeping a thriving herb garden. Understanding the benefits of mulching, selecting the correct materials, and adopting efficient weed control strategies will allow you to create an ideal environment for your herbs to thrive. A well-kept garden not only produces healthy and flavorful herbs, but it also requires less upkeep in the long run. Embrace these methods to have a healthy herb garden all year!

ORGANIC PEST MANAGEMENT.

Maintaining a productive herb garden requires keeping your plants healthy and pest-free. Chemical pesticides can be helpful, but they also pose threats to your health, the environment, and beneficial insects. Organic pest management is a safer, more sustainable option that prioritizes prevention, natural solutions, and biodiversity. In this chapter, we'll look at various organic pest management options to help you safeguard your herb garden while keeping its ecological balance.

Understanding Pests

Common Herbal Pests

Identifying common pests is the first step towards efficient management. Here are some common pests that could infect your herb garden:

Aphids are tiny, soft-bodied insects that drain sap from plants, causing wilting and stunted growth.
- Spider Mites: Microscopic pests that form fine webs on the undersides of leaves, causing yellowing and leaf fall.
- Whiteflies are little, white flying insects that feed

on plant sap, weakening plants and perhaps spreading illnesses.
- Caterpillars: Moth and butterfly larvae that, if not handled, can rapidly defoliate your plants.

Example: Aphids are commonly observed collecting on the fragile young growth of basil and parsley, making early detection critical.

Preventive Measures

Creating A Healthy Environment

Prevention is the most effective technique for organic pest management. Here are some basic measures for maintaining a healthy herb garden:

- Diverse Planting: Use a variety of herbs and flowers to attract beneficial insects, which can aid in pest control.
- Healthy Soil: Use organic compost and fertilizers to keep the soil healthy, resulting in robust, resilient plants that can endure pest attacks.
- Companion Planting: Pairing specific plants can help prevent pests. For example, planting marigolds near plants can deter aphids and nematodes.

Example: Interplanting nasturtiums beside your herbs can keep aphids away from your more costly plants.

Organic Pest Control Strategies

Natural Remedies

When prevention isn't adequate, natural solutions can efficiently manage insect populations:

- Insecticidal Soaps: These soaps suffocate soft-bodied insects such as aphids and spider mites while not harming beneficial insects.
- Neem Oil: Neem oil, derived from neem tree seeds, affects pests' life cycles and functions as a repellant.
- Diatomaceous Earth: This natural powder is good against crawling insects, dehydrating them on contact.

Example: Spraying a diluted solution of neem oil on your basil can help prevent pests while not damaging the plant.

Beneficial Insects

Promoting beneficial insects in your garden is a fantastic technique for natural pest management.

- Ladybugs: These beetles eat aphids and other tiny pests, making them valuable garden companions.
- Lacewing larvae eat a lot of aphids, spider mites,

and other pests.
- Parasitic Wasps: These small wasps lay their eggs within problem insects, eventually reducing their numbers.

Example: Planting flowers such as dill and fennel can attract ladybugs and lacewings, resulting in a natural pest control system.

Monitoring and managing infestations

Regular Inspections

Regular monitoring of your garden is essential for the early detection of pest issues.

- Visual Inspection: Examine the leaves and stems of your herbs for evidence of pest activity or damage.
- Sticky traps: Place yellow sticky traps near your plants to capture flying pests such as whiteflies and fungus gnats.

Example: A weekly trip through your herb garden might help you identify any pest problems before they worsen.

Remove Infested Plants

If you discover a significant infestation, consider

removing the damaged plant to avoid further spread:

- Isolation: To prevent pests from spreading to healthy plants, isolate the affected plant.
- Companion Planting: Consider swapping out the affected plant with a pest-resistant cultivar.

Example: If a pot of oregano becomes infested with spider mites, it can be removed and replaced with a more resistant plant, such as rosemary, to help keep your garden healthy.

Organic pest management is a long-term technique that prioritizes the health of both your herb garden and the environment. Understanding pests, taking preventive steps, using natural therapies, and encouraging helpful insects are all ways to effectively protect your herbs from pest damage. Adopt the organic growing concept and enjoy a thriving, healthy herb garden that not only produces delectable ingredients but also helps to maintain a balanced ecology.

HARVESTING AND PRESERVING HERBS

When and How to Harvest.

Harvesting herbs at the appropriate time and with the proper techniques can considerably improve the flavor and potency of your culinary creations. Knowing when to harvest your herbs not only enhances their flavor, but it also promotes continued development and healthy plants. In this chapter, we will look at the best methods for harvesting your herbs, including the optimum timing, procedures, and recommendations for getting the most out of your harvest.

When To Harvest

Timing is important.

The timing of your herb harvest has a significant impact on the flavor, aroma, and quality of your herbs. Here are some important considerations to consider.

- Growth Stage: Harvest herbs at their peak growth, usually immediately before they blossom. This is when they have the most flavor and scent.
- Time of Day: Herbs are best harvested in the morning after the dew has dried but before the heat of the day. This helps to preserve the essential oils

and tastes.
- Weather weather: Avoid harvesting in moist weather or after heavy rain, since this might result in mold and spoiling.

Example: Basil is best gathered in the morning, just before it flowers, to capture its bright flavor and essential oils.

How to Harvest

Techniques for various herbs

Different herbs may necessitate distinct harvesting practices to ensure optimal flavor and plant health. Here are a few effective methods:

- Pinching: For herbs such as basil, mint, and oregano, pinch off the tips of the stems just above the leaf nodes. This promotes bushier growth while preventing legginess.
- Cut: To cut stems of herbs like thyme and rosemary, use sharp scissors or pruning shears. Cut just above a group of leaves to promote regrowth.
- pulling: For herbs such as chives or garlic chives, carefully pluck the entire plant or clip the leaves at the base to promote new growth.

Example: When collecting chives, cut them at the base, leaving approximately an inch above the earth for regrowth.

Harvesting Quantities

It's crucial to know how much to harvest to keep your plants healthy and fruitful.

- Regular Harvesting: To avoid overharvesting, harvest about one-third of a culinary herb plant at a time.
- Seasonal Considerations: Harvest more generously throughout the early growing season, then reduce harvesting as the season develops to allow for restocking.

Example: If your parsley plant is flourishing, you can safely harvest a large amount early in the season, but you should cut back as fall approaches to ensure winter survival.

Postharvest Care

Cleaning and Preparing Herbs

After you've picked your herbs, you must clean and prepare them properly:

- Rinse To eliminate dirt and insects from your plants, gently rinse them under cool running water. Use a salad spinner to remove any extra moisture.

- Drying: Pat the herbs dry with a clean towel or paper towel to prevent moisture from forming mold while in storage.

Example: After picking cilantro, gently rinse it and completely dry it to keep it fresher longer in your refrigerator.

Storing Fresh Herbs

Storing your freshly collected herbs properly helps extend their shelf life and preserve their flavor:

- Refrigeration: Place fresh herbs, such as basil and parsley, in a jar with water, cover with a plastic bag, and refrigerate.
- Freezing: For long-term storage, cut herbs and set them in ice cube trays filled with water or oil before freezing for later use.

Example: By freezing chopped basil in ice cube trays, you can simply add fresh flavor to soups and sauces throughout the winter.

Harvesting your herbs at the right time and using the proper techniques guarantees that you get the maximum flavor and scent. By paying attention to development stages, scheduling, and proper harvesting procedures, you can keep your herb plants healthy while increasing your culinary potential. With these abilities, you'll be able to reap the benefits of your labor and include fresh herbs into your meals for years to come.

DRYING AND STORING HERBS

Drying herbs is one of the oldest and most successful ways to keep their flavor, aroma, and therapeutic characteristics. By eliminating moisture from your herbs, you may extend their shelf life and keep a cache of homegrown flavors on hand even during the off-season. In this chapter, we'll look at different ways for drying herbs, how to properly store them, and how to use your preserved herbs in the kitchen.

Why Dry Herbs?

Advantages of Drying

Drying herbs not only helps preserve their flavors, but it also has several other benefits:

- Extended Shelf Life: When stored properly, dried herbs can survive for months or even years, making them an ideal way to enjoy your garden's abundance all year.
- room-Saving: Dried herbs take up far less room than fresh ones, making them easier to store and organize.

- Concentration of Flavor: Drying herbs enhances their flavors, making them a more robust addition to your cuisine.

Example: A tablespoon of dried basil might have a stronger flavor than a tablespoon of fresh basil because of the concentration of oils and chemicals throughout the drying process.

Methods to Dry Herbs

Selecting the Right Method

There are various effective methods for drying herbs, and the ideal one depends on the type of herb and the resources you have.

1. Air drying is ideal for herbs with low moisture content, such as thyme, rosemary, and sage.
Steps: - Gather stems and knot them together using twine or string.
- Hang them upside down in a warm, dry, well-ventilated room out of direct sunshine.
- Let dry for 1 to 3 weeks, monitoring for dryness at regular intervals.

2. Oven Drying: - Ideal for rapid drying, especially in humid conditions.
- Steps: - Preheat oven to lowest setting (approx. 170°F/77°C).

- Arrange the herbs on a baking sheet in a single layer.
- Place them in the oven with the door slightly ajar to let moisture out.
- Check every 30 minutes and remove when crispy.

3. Dehydrator: - Effectively dries huge amounts of herbs fast and efficiently.
- Steps:
- Arrange the herbs on the dehydrator trays in a single layer.
- Set the temperature following the manufacturer's recommendations (typically between 95°F and 115°F).
- Dry for 1–4 hours, depending on the herb and dehydrator type.

4. Microwave Drying: - Fastest process, ideal for small amounts.
Steps: - Place herbs between two paper towels.
- Microwave at low power in 30-second intervals until completely dry.
Allow to cool before storing.

Example: If you're in a hurry, the microwave method can dry fresh mint in a matter of minutes, making it ideal for your favorite tea!

Storing Dried Herbs

Best Storage Practices

Dried herbs must be stored properly to maintain their quality and flavor. Here are a few tips:

To protect dried herbs from air and moisture, store them in airtight containers such as glass jars, metal tins, or vacuum-sealed bags.
- Labeled Containers: To ensure freshness, clearly label your containers with the herb name and drying date.
- Cool and Dark Place: To keep your herbs fresh, store them in a cold, dark cabinet or pantry.

Example: A labeled glass jar of dried oregano can help organize your spice closet while keeping the herb fresh and delicious.

Shelf Life of Dried Herbs

While dried herbs can persist for months or years, their strength progressively decreases with time. Below are some general guidelines:

- Whole Leaves: Dried whole leaves can last between one and three years.
- Ground or crushed herbs: These normally last 6-12 months until their flavor fades.
- Check for freshness: Always verify the aroma and flavor of your dried herbs before using. If they smell

stale or lack flavor, replace them.

Using Dried Herbs for Cooking

Flavoring Your Dishes

Dried herbs can be used in several culinary applications:

- Seasoning: Add dried herbs to soups, stews, sauces, and marinades to boost taste.
- Infusing: Create tasty infusions by combining dry herbs with oils or vinegar.
- Baking tip: Add dried herbs to bread or savory baked items for a fragrant twist.

Example: A sprinkling of dried thyme may improve a simple chicken broth, giving it depth and richness.

Drying and storing herbs is a simple but efficient approach to reap the benefits of your efforts long after the growing season is over. You may enjoy the flavors of your herb garden all year by using the best drying method, properly storing your herbs, and incorporating them into your meals. Learn how to dry and preserve your own herbs, and use them to enhance your culinary creations.

MAKING HERBAL INFUSIONS AND TEAS.

Herbal infusions and teas are a delicious way to enjoy the flavors and health benefits of your garden produce. Whether you want a relaxing evening drink or a refreshing afternoon pick-me-up, herbal teas can bring both pleasure and wellness. In this chapter, we'll look at how to make herbal infusions, what herbs you can use, and how to tailor your brews to your preferences and health needs.

Understanding Herbal Infusions and Teas.

What are herbal infusions?

Herbal infusions are made by steeping herbs in boiling water to extract their flavor, aroma, and medicinal ingredients. This procedure may be as easy or as sophisticated as you like, making it suitable for everyone, from newbie herbalists to seasoned tea connoisseurs.

- Infusion vs. Decoction: - Infusion: Use hot water to extract tastes and oils from delicate leaves, flowers, and stems, such as chamomile and mint.
- Decoction: Simmering harder components of plants, such as roots and seeds, extracts their tastes (e.g., ginger, cinnamon).

Example: Chamomile flowers form a calming infusion, whilst ginger root takes a stew to release its lively flavor.

Selecting Your Herbs

Popular Herbs for Infusions and Teas

You can make wonderful infusions with a wide variety of herbs. Here are a few popular options:

- Peppermint: Energizing and refreshing; excellent for digestion.
- Lemon Balm: Calming and energizing; ideal for stress reduction.
- Lavender: Soothing and aromatic; promotes relaxation and sleep.
- Rooibos: Naturally caffeine-free, high in antioxidants, and ideal as a base for herbal blends.

Example: A combination of peppermint and lemon balm produces a pleasant tea that is both relaxing and energetic.

How to Prepare Herbal Infusions and Teas

Step-by-Step Guidelines

Follow these easy steps to make your herbal infusion or tea:

1. Select Your Herbs: - Choose fresh or dried herbs

based on desired flavor and impact.

2. To measure the herbs, use 1 to 2 teaspoons of dry herbs or 2 to 3 teaspoons of fresh herbs per cup of water.

3. Heat Water: Bring filtered water to boil. After boiling the water to roughly 190°F (88°C), let it cool for a minute before adding delicate herbs.

4. Steep Herbs: - Place the herbs in a tea infuser, or directly into a teapot or cup. Pour the hot water on the herbs.
- Cover and steep for 5–10 minutes, depending on the strength you like.

5. Strain and Serve: - Remove herbs with a strainer or infuser. Enjoy your herbal infusion simply or with honey, lemon, or other flavors to taste.

Example: Steeping dried lavender flowers for 7 minutes yields a fragrant infusion that can be served warm or chilled.

Customizing your infusions

Creating Unique Flavor Profiles.

Experimenting with different herbs allows you to build your own mixtures. Here are some suggestions to customize your herbal teas:

- Combine Herbs: Combine herbs to boost flavor and benefits. Chamomile, for example, works well with lemon balm to promote relaxation.
- Add Citrus: A slice of lemon or orange can brighten the flavor and provide a refreshing touch.
- Spice Up: Spices such as cinnamon and ginger can be used to provide warmth and additional health advantages.

Example: To make a hot chai infusion, combine rooibos, cinnamon, ginger, and cardamom.

Storing herbal teas

Keeping Your Infusions Fresh.

If you enjoy producing big batches of herbal tea, appropriate storage is critical to ensuring freshness.

- Store in airtight containers: To keep dried herbs fresh, store them in dark glass jars or airtight containers.
- Label and date: To ensure freshness, clearly label your containers with the herb's name and date.

Example: A labeled jar of dried peppermint can be a welcome addition to your tea collection, ready to brew whenever you want a refreshing drink.

Making herbal infusions and teas is a simple yet satisfying way to enjoy the flavors and benefits of your garden plants. With a little imagination and experimentation, you can make delectable blends tailored to your preferences and wellness requirements. Whether you drink herbal tea alone for a moment of quiet or with friends, these infusions can help you feel better overall.

CREATING HERBAL TINCTURES AND EXTRACTS.

Herbal tinctures and extracts are effective strategies to harness the therapeutic benefits of herbs while making them more accessible for everyday usage. These concentrated solutions can improve health, promote wellness, and function as natural cures in your home apothecary. In this chapter, we'll learn about tinctures and extracts, how they're made, and how to use them safely and successfully.

Understanding Herbal Tinctures and Extracts

What is a tincture?

A tincture is a concentrated liquid form of herbal medicine created by soaking herbs in alcohol or another solvent. The extraction procedure extracts the active components, tastes, and fragrances, producing a strong herbal solution.

- Alcohol Tinctures: Typically produced with high-proof alcohol (such as vodka), which removes both water-soluble and alcohol-soluble components.
- Glycerin Tinctures: Made with vegetable glycerin, ideal for individuals who want alcohol-free choices.

Example: Echinacea tincture can boost immunological function, whereas valerian root tincture can encourage relaxation.

What is an Extract?

Herbal extracts are similar to tinctures, but they can be prepared using a variety of solvents such as water, vinegar, or glycerin. Extracts are often less concentrated than tinctures and can be used in cooking, herbal treatments, or as flavorings.

- Herbal extracts: These can be made with either fresh or dried herbs, depending on your preferences.

Example: Vanilla extract, which is often used in baking, is a herbal extract created by steeping vanilla beans in alcohol.

Making Herbal Tinctures

Step-by-Step Procedure

Making a herbal tincture is a rewarding and simple process. This is how you do it:

1. Choose Your Herb: - Choose dried or fresh herbs with proven health benefits.

2. Gather supplies:
To prepare, you'll need a clean glass jar with a tight-fitting lid and at least 80 percent alcohol.
- A dark glass dropper bottle for storing.
- cheesecloth or a fine mesh sieve.

3. Prepare Herbs: - Chop fresh or smash dried herbs to enhance surface area for extraction.
- Fill the jar with the prepared herbs, leaving some room at the top.

4. Add the Alcohol: - Pour enough alcohol to completely submerge the herbs, leaving no air pockets.

5. Seal and Shake: - Tightly seal the container and shake vigorously to combine the herbs and alcohol.

6. Step: - Store the jar in a cold, dark area for 4–6 weeks. Shake lightly every few days to aid in the extraction process.

7. Strain and Store: After steeping, strain the mixture through cheesecloth or fine mesh strainer

into a clean bottle. Label the bottle with the herb's name and date.

Example: An elderberry tincture can be made by steeping dried elderberries in alcohol for many weeks, yielding a potent immune-boosting medicine.

Producing Herbal Extracts

Simple Steps for Extracts

Herbal extracts are as simple to make and can be a useful addition to your kitchen. Here's how to make a basic herbal extract.

1. Select Your Herb: - Choose herbs for their flavor or health benefits.

2. Gather materials:
You will need a glass jar.
- Water, vinegar, or glycerin (for the solvent)
- Cheesecloth or strainer.

3. Prepare the Herbs: - Crush or chop the herbs to release vital oils and tastes.

4. Combine and store: Place the herbs in a jar and cover with your desired solvent. Seal tightly.

5. Infuse: - Store the mixture in a cold, dark area for

2–4 weeks. Shake it occasionally.

6. Strain and Bottle: - After infusing, strain the mixture into a dark glass bottle and label it for future use.

Example: Basil extract can be generated by soaking fresh basil leaves in vinegar, which adds flavor to salad dressings and marinades.

Safety and Usage

Tips for Using Tinctures and Extracts

When utilizing herbal tinctures and extracts, keep the following things in mind:

- Dosage: Begin with a tiny dose (usually 1-2 droppers of tincture) and monitor your body's response.
- Consultation: If you are pregnant, nursing, or taking medication, see a doctor before using herbal tinctures or extracts.
- Storage: Keep tinctures and extracts in a cold, dark place to maintain their potency.

Example: A few drops of lavender tincture can be added to your nighttime routine to promote relaxation, but start with a lesser amount to see how it works.

Making herbal tinctures and extracts is a rewarding method to maximize the power of your homegrown herbs. With a little preparation and patience, you can reap the advantages of herbal treatments in concentrated form. Whether you want to boost your immune system, flavor your food, or improve your wellness regimen, tinctures and extracts can be important allies. Dive into the realm of herbal concoctions to maximize the benefits of your garden's bounty!

USING MEDICINAL HERBS FOR HEALTH AND WELLNESS

Herbal remedies for Common Ailments

Including herbal treatments in your wellness routine can be a natural and effective way to treat common problems. Medicinal herbs have been used for generations to improve health and well-being, ranging from calming stomach disorders to stress relief. This chapter will look at numerous herbal cures for common ailments, providing practical knowledge and examples to help you on your journey to natural health.

Understanding Herbal Remedies.

Herbal treatments are made from plant leaves, flowers, roots, and stems and can be taken in a variety of formats such as teas, tinctures, capsules, or extracts. Each plant has distinct qualities and benefits, making it appropriate for a variety of health conditions.

Common Ailments with Herbal Solutions

1. Digestive Issues

- Peppermint: Peppermint tea is known for its ability to relieve digestive discomfort, such as bloating,

gas, and indigestion.
- How to Use: Brew peppermint leaves in hot water and drink after each meal.
- Here's an example: A cup of peppermint tea can be soothing after a big dinner.

- Ginger: This warming herb relieves nausea and motion sickness.
- How To Use: Grate fresh ginger and steep in boiling water to make tea.
- Here's an example: Ginger tea is a popular treatment for morning sickness during pregnancy.

2: Stress and Anxiety

- Chamomile: Chamomile tea, known for its relaxing effects, will help you relax and sleep better.
- How to Use: Soak dried chamomile flowers in hot water for 5–10 minutes.
- Here's an example: A cup of chamomile tea before bed might help you relax and prepare for a good night's sleep.

- Lavender: The aroma of lavender has been shown to lower anxiety and stress levels.
- How to Use: Place lavender essential oil in a diffuser or make a soothing herbal sachet.
- Here's an example: Inhaling lavender oil might help to create a peaceful environment for relaxation.

3: Cold and Flu

- Echinacea: Echinacea is commonly used to enhance the immune system and may help shorten the duration of colds.
- How To Use: Take echinacea pills or make a tincture.
- Here's an example: Echinacea can be especially effective when taken at the first sign of a cold.

- Elderberry: This berry is high in antioxidants and may help lessen flu symptoms and minimize sickness duration.
- How to Use: Take elderberry syrup or brew a tea with dried elderberries.
- Here's an example: Elderberry syrup is a popular alternative for youngsters throughout the cold and flu season.

4. Skin Conditions

- Calendula: Calendula, which is known for its anti-inflammatory and healing characteristics, can help with minor cuts and skin irritations.
- How To Use: Apply calendula-infused oil or ointment to affected areas.
- Here's an example: Calendula cream can be used to relieve diaper rash in newborns.

- Aloe Vera: This succulent is well-known for its

capacity to moisturize and heal the skin.
- How to Use: Apply fresh aloe vera gel straight from the plant to burnt or irritated skin.
- Here's an example: Aloe vera is a popular cure for sunburn relief.

Safety Considerations.

While herbal medicines can be effective, they should be used with caution:

- Consult with a Healthcare Provider: Before using herbal treatments, consult a healthcare practitioner, especially if you are pregnant, nursing, or taking any drugs.
- Know Your Dosage: Because herbs have significant effects, it is important to follow suggested amounts.
- sensitivities: Be cautious if you have any sensitivities to specific herbs.

Herbal medicines provide a wealth of natural treatments to common problems, allowing you to take control of your health in a holistic manner. By including these herbs into your wellness routine, you can reap their benefits while also developing a stronger connection with nature. Experiment with various herbs to see what works best for you, and embrace the path to health and wellness via the power of medicinal herbs.

RECIPES FOR HERBAL SALVE AND BALM

Herbal salves and balms are flexible therapies that use medicinal herbs' healing abilities to provide soothing relief for a variety of skin diseases while also encouraging general health. These natural remedies are simple to make at home, requiring only a few ingredients and steps. In this chapter, we'll look at how to make herbal salves and balms, as well as recipes for various requirements, so you may make your own healing treatments right in your kitchen.

Understanding Herbal Salves and Balms

What is a salve?

A salve is a thick, ointment-like solution that soothes, heals, and protects the skin. Salves are frequently made up of a combination of herbal-infused oils, beeswax, and essential oils, which act as a barrier to moisture and promote healing.

What is a balm?

A balm is comparable to a salve, but with a softer consistency. Balms are frequently created with oils and butters, such as shea or cocoa butter, which make them excellent for nourishing and hydrating the skin.

Advantages of Using Herbal Salves and Balms

- Natural substances: Herbal products contain plant-based substances that are soft on the skin and free of synthetic chemicals.
- Targeted Relief: Salves and balms can be designed to address specific skin issues, such as dry skin or small injuries.
- Easy to Make: With just a few basic components, you may make excellent treatments at home.

Recipes for Herbal Salve and Balm

1. Healing Herbal Salve.

Ingredients:
- 1 cup olive oil (or carrier oil of your preference)
- 1/2 cup dried herbs (Calendula, Chamomile, or Lavender)
- 1/4 cup beeswax pellets.
- Optional: Essential oils (e.g., tea tree, lavender) for further benefits

Instructions: 1. To infuse the oil, put olive oil and dried herbs in a double boiler. Heat on low for 2-3 hours to let the herbs infuse.
2. Strain the Mixture: After infusing, strain the oil through cheesecloth or a fine mesh strainer to remove the herbs.

3. Add Beeswax: Return the infused oil to the double boiler, then add the beeswax pellets and stir until melted.
4. Pour and cool: Remove from the heat, add essential oils if preferred, and pour into clean jars or tins. Let cool completely before sealing.

Example: This healing salve can be used on minor cuts, scrapes, or dry skin to provide soothing comfort and promote recovery.

 2. Soothing Lavender Balm

Ingredients:
- Use 1/2 cup coconut oil and 1/2 cup shea butter. Use 1/4 cup beeswax pellets and 20 drops lavender essential oil.

Instructions:
1. Melt the Base: In a double boiler, heat the coconut oil, shea butter, and beeswax. Heat until everything is melted and thoroughly combined.
2. Add Essential Oil: Remove from heat and whisk in lavender essential oil, which has relaxing characteristics.
3. pour and set: Pour the mixture into containers and let it cool until firm.

Example: This lavender balm is ideal for hydrating dry skin and can also be used as a soothing moisturizer before bedtime.

3: Herbal Muscle Rub

Ingredients:
- One cup olive oil.
Ingredients: 1/2 cup dried arnica flowers, 1/4 cup beeswax, and 10 drops of peppermint essential oil.
- Ten drops of eucalyptus essential oil

Instructions: 1. To prepare an infused oil, heat olive oil and arnica flowers in a double boiler for 2-3 hours.
2. To remove the flowers, strain the oil.
3. Combine with Beeswax: Return the infused oil to the double boiler, add the beeswax, and melt them together.
4. Add Essential Oils: Once melted, remove from heat and incorporate the essential oils.
5. Pour and Cool: Transfer to jars and allow to set.

Example: This herbal muscle massage is great for relieving tight muscles and tension after exercise.

Tips for Success

- Storage: Keep your salves and balms in a cold, dark place to extend their shelf life. Jars that are properly sealed can last a year or more.
- LABELING: Label each container with the name

and date of preparation so that it may be easily identified.
- Patch Test: Before using a new salve or balm, conduct a patch test on a small area of skin to rule out any adverse reactions.

Making your own herbal salves and balms is a satisfying way to incorporate the healing power of plants into your daily life. With simple ingredients and straightforward methods, you may create bespoke cures that address your specific health needs. Learn the art of herbal preparation and enjoy the benefits of using nature's gifts to promote wellness and healing in your own home.

CREATING YOUR OWN HERBAL FIRST AID KIT

A well-stocked herbal first aid kit can be a great tool for treating minor injuries and illnesses at home. By combining medicinal herbs, you can produce a natural alternative to traditional first aid materials. This chapter will walk you through the essential components of a herbal first aid kit, including recipes and how to use these natural medications efficiently.

Why Make An Herbal First Aid Kit?

- Natural Remedies: Herbal first aid kits offer plant-

based treatments for common ailments, decreasing dependency on synthetic drugs.
- Preparation: Having herbal treatments on hand can save time and money in an emergency, allowing you to address minor issues swiftly.
- Empowerment: Making your own kit offers you more control over your health and a better awareness of the therapeutic powers of plants.

Essential Ingredients for Your Herbal First Aid Kit

1. Herbal Treatments for Common Ailments

- Calendula Salve: Calendula salve is known for its anti-inflammatory and healing characteristics and can be used to treat cuts, scrapes, and rashes.
- Arnica Gel: This herbal medicine relieves bruises, sprains, and muscle aches.
- Peppermint Tea: This relaxing tea can assist with headaches, nausea, and intestinal pain.

2. Basic First Aid Supplies

- Bandages and Gauze: These items are essential for wound coverage and infection prevention.
- Antiseptic Wipes: Use herbal-infused wipes with witch hazel or tea tree oil to provide natural antiseptic characteristics.
- Thermometer: To monitor fevers and provide

proper care.

Recipes for Herbal First Aid Kits

1. Calendula Salve

Ingredients:
- 1 cup olive oil (or carrier oil of your preference)
- 1/2 cup dried calendula flowers.
- 1/4 cup beeswax pellets.

Instructions: 1. In a double boiler, blend olive oil and calendula flowers to infuse oil. Heat on low for around 2-3 hours.
2. Strain and Add Beeswax: Strain the oil and return it to the double boiler. Melt the beeswax.
3. Cool and Store Pour into tiny containers and let cool.

Usage: Apply the salve to small wounds, scratches, and rashes to get rapid relief.

2: Arnica Gel

Ingredients:
- 1/2 cup dried arnica flowers.
- One cup carrier oil (such as olive or coconut oil)
- 1/4 cup aloe vera gel - 10 drops essential oil (such as lavender or peppermint)

Instructions:
1. Infuse Oil: Cook arnica flowers in carrier oil over a double boiler for 2-3 hours.
2. Strain: Combine the oil, aloe vera gel, and essential oil.
3. Storage: Transfer the mixture to a squeeze bottle or jar.

Usage: Apply on bruises, sprains, and aching muscles to provide comfort.

Tips for Putting Together Your Herbal First Aid Kit

- Storage: Choose a durable container that is easy to transport and protects your materials from moisture and light. A tiny backpack or plastic tote works great.
- Labeling: Make sure to clearly mark each herbal cure with its name and intended usage for easy identification during an emergency.
- Regular updates: Regularly check your kit for expired goods and restock supplies as needed.

Making your own herbal first aid pack allows you to treat minor health conditions naturally and effectively. By incorporating important herbal treatments and basic first aid supplies, you can equip yourself and your family with the resources they require for health and wellness. Accept the healing power of herbs and prepare for a better, more resilient tomorrow.

INCORPORATING HERBS INTO DAILY LIFE

Integrating medicinal herbs into your daily routine can improve your overall health and wellness while also providing natural solutions to a variety of everyday difficulties. From infusions to gastronomic treats, the options are limitless. This chapter looks at practical ways to include herbs into your daily routine, making them an essential component of your health and well-being.

Advantages of Using Herbs Daily

- Promotes Wellness: Using herbs on a regular basis can help increase immunity, improve digestion, and elevate mood.
- Natural Flavoring: Herbs offer flavor to foods without the use of harmful additives or excessive salt.
- Sustainable Living: Growing and using herbs promotes a more sustainable living by linking you to nature.

Practical Ways to Integrate Herbs into Daily Life

1. Herbal infusions and teas

- Begin Your Day Right: Drink a cup of herbal tea, such as chamomile for relaxation or peppermint for digestion.
- Hydration Boost: To add a refreshing twist to hydration, infuse water with fresh herbs like mint, basil, or lemon balm.

Example: Make a delightful mint tea by steeping fresh mint leaves in boiling water for 5–10 minutes. If desired, add honey for sweetness.

2. Culinary Application

- Seasoning Your Dishes: Use herbs like thyme, rosemary, or oregano in your cooking to boost flavor and nutrients.
- Salads and Dressings: Fresh herbs such as parsley, cilantro, or basil can be chopped and mixed into salads or homemade dressings to enhance flavor.

Example: Make a tasty herb vinaigrette by combining olive oil, vinegar, fresh herbs, garlic, salt, and pepper.

3. Herbal Supplements

- Capsules and Extracts: Use herbal capsules or extracts for specific advantages, such as

ashwagandha for stress reduction or elderberry for immune support.
- Smoothie Boost: To add a nutritional boost to your morning smoothie, try powdered herbs like spirulina, maca, or matcha.

Example: Make a nutritious green smoothie by blending spinach, banana, almond milk, a teaspoon of spirulina powder, and a handful of ice.

4. Aromatherapy and Herbal Remedies.

- Essential Oils: Incorporate essential oils into your daily routine by diffusing them throughout your home or adding them to your bath for a relaxing soak.
- Topical Applications: Use herbal-infused oils or balms for skin care, muscle relaxation, or as a natural scent substitute.

Example: Make a relaxing aromatherapy combination by combining lavender essential oil and a carrier oil and applying it to pulse points.

Tips for Success

- Grow Your Own: Begin a small herb garden, either indoors or outdoors, to have fresh herbs available for daily usage.
- Experiment and Learn: Try different herbs and

recipes to see which ones work best for your health and taste preferences.
- Listen to Your Body: Pay attention to how your body reacts to various herbs and adjust your dosage accordingly.

Incorporating herbs into your daily routine is a gratifying and engaging experience that promotes health, wellness, and a stronger connection with nature. By experimenting with herbs in a variety of ways, from culinary pleasures to relaxing teas and essential oils, you can improve your health while enjoying the many flavors and advantages that these plants provide. Accept the power of herbs and allow them to change your everyday routine into a holistic health journey.

ADVANCED HERBAL GARDENING TECHNIQUES.

Propagation Methods: Cuttings and Divisions

Propagation is the art and science of growing new plants from existing ones, and it's a necessary skill for any herbal gardener who wants to extend their garden or share their favorite herbs with others. Cuttings and divisions are two of the most successful and popular ways to propagate herbs. This chapter will delve into these strategies, offering step-by-step instructions, success tips, and examples to assist you in mastering the art of propagation.

Benefits of Propagation

- Cost-Effective: Growing your own herbs saves money over purchasing new plants from a nursery.
- Genetic Consistency: Using cuttings assures that the new plants are genetically identical to their parents, keeping beneficial characteristics.
- Garden Expansion: Dividing established plants helps you to grow your garden with little work and time.

Propagation Methods

1. Propagation via Cuttings

Cuttings are pieces of stems or leaves removed from a parent plant that can root and sprout into a new plant. This approach is particularly effective for several herbs, including basil, mint, and rosemary.

Steps to Take Cuttings:

- Select the Right Plant: Choose a healthy, strong plant to take cuttings from, preferably during the growing season.
- Choose the Right Cut: Choose a stem that is at least 4-6 inches long and contains many leaf nodes. Softwood cuttings are best in the spring and early summer, but hardwood cuttings are better in the late fall or winter.
- Prepare the Cutting: - Use clean, sharp scissors or a knife to cut just below a node (where leaves emerge).
- Remove the lower leaves to expose the nodes, leaving a few leaves on top for photosynthesis.
- Rooting Hormone (Optional): Dip the cut end in rooting hormone to promote rapid root growth; however, many herbs root successfully without it.
- Plant the Cutting: Place the cutting in a pot with moist potting mix, burying the node in the dirt.
- Create a Humid Environment: Cover the pot with a plastic bag or a clear plastic dome to keep humidity in while removing roots.
- Water and Light: Keep the soil moist but not

waterlogged, and set the pot somewhere with bright, indirect light.

Example: Try propagating basil by taking 4-inch cuttings, immersing them in water, then transplanting them to soil once they have roots.

 2. Propagation by Division

Division is the process of dividing an established herb plant into smaller pieces, each with their own roots and shoots. This approach is widely used with perennial herbs such as chives, thyme, and oregano.

Steps for Dividing Plants:

- Choose the Right Time: Most herb plants are best divided in early spring or fall, when they are not actively developing.
- Prepare the Tools: Gather a spade, garden fork, or shovel for digging, as well as pots or garden space for each separated part.
- Dug Up the Plant: Dig carefully around the plant to avoid disturbing the roots, then gently take it from the earth.
- Separate the Roots. Using your hands or tools, gently separate the root clusters. Each portion should contain roots and branches. Aim for pieces with at least a couple inches in diameter.
- Replant or Pot Up: Replant the separated parts

immediately, making sure they are the same depth as previously. Water thoroughly to help settle the dirt.
- Care for the New Plants: Monitor the divided plants' water needs and keep them out of direct sunlight until they establish.

Example: To divide a mature chive plant, carefully peel apart the tight clumps of roots and replant each section in well-prepared soil.

Strategies for Successful Propagation

- Choose Healthy Parent Plants: To promote vigorous new growth, only take cuttings and divisions from healthy, disease-free plants.
- Be Patient: Rooting cuttings might take time (usually a few weeks), so be patient and provide the ideal conditions for success.
- Identify and label new plants: Keep track of the types you propagate by identifying your new plants with their names and dates.

Mastering propagation techniques such as cuttings and divisions is a satisfying way to improve your herbal garden while saving money and assuring a steady supply of your favorite herbs. Understanding the techniques and following the steps provided in this chapter will help you become an expert herbal propagator.

GROWING HERBS IN CONTAINERS

Growing herbs in containers is a useful and satisfying option for both new and seasoned gardeners. Whether you have limited space, poor soil quality, or simply want the freedom to move your plants, container gardening has several advantages. In this chapter, we'll look at the fundamentals of container gardening, such as the best containers, appropriate herbs, soil preparation, and care practices to guarantee your herbs grow.

Benefits of Container Gardening

- Space Efficiency: Container gardening is perfect for small spaces, balconies, or patios, allowing everyone to enjoy fresh herbs.
- Mobility: Containers can be moved to take advantage of the best sunlight, shade, or protection from bad weather.
- Soil Control: You have control over the soil quality, ensuring optimal growing conditions customized to your herbs' individual requirements.
- Pest Management: Container gardening can help minimize the spread of soil-borne pests and illnesses.

Selecting the Right Containers

When it comes to growing herbs in containers,

choosing the right pots is essential. Here are some important considerations to consider.

1: Material

- Terracotta: Excellent for drainage and breathability, although they dry out rapidly, necessitating more frequent watering.
- Plastic: Lightweight and inexpensive, plastic containers retain moisture well but may lack appropriate airflow.
- Ceramic: Ceramic pots are both attractive and durable, and they frequently include a glaze that helps retain moisture. However, they can be heavy.

2. Size

- Most herbs require pots with a diameter of at least 6-12 inches. Larger pots can hold several plants or larger species, such as basil or rosemary.

3. Drainage

- Make sure containers have drainage holes to avoid waterlogging, which can lead to root rot. If you're using beautiful pots without drainage, use them as exterior pots and place smaller pots inside.

Best Herbs for Container Gardening

Many herbs grow in containers. Here are a few popular choices:

- Basil: Prefers warm weather and can thrive in a sunny location.
- Mint: Grows quickly, making it excellent for use in containers to minimize spreading.
- Chives: A hardy herb that grows well in containers and requires little maintenance.
- Thyme: A low-growing herb that thrives in smaller pots and requires little maintenance.
- Rosemary: A drought-tolerant herb that benefits from being kept in a container to improve drainage.

Soil Preparation for Container Herbs

- Potting Mix: Use a high-quality potting mix that is specifically designed for container planting. This mixture is lighter and drains more efficiently than garden soil.
- Additives: Use perlite or vermiculite to increase aeration and drainage, or mix in organic compost to replenish the soil with nutrients.

Techniques for Container Herbs

1: Watering

- Frequency: Container herbs require more frequent watering than garden-planted herbs since they dry

up more quickly.
- Method: Thoroughly rinse with water until it drains from the bottom. Avoid leaving the soil moist.

2: Sunlight

- Most herbs require full sun, so position containers in areas with at least 6-8 hours of sunlight every day. However, be aware of the severe heat and provide some shade if necessary.

3. Fertilization

- Frequency: Apply a balanced liquid fertilizer to container herbs every 4-6 weeks during the growing season.
- Organic Options: Consider using organic fertilizers such as fish emulsion or seaweed extract to add nutrients without the use of chemicals.

Example: Establishing a Container Herb Garden

1. Select Your Herbs: Combine a variety of your favorite herbs, such as basil, parsley, and chives.
2. Choose Containers: Use 10-inch terracotta pots with drainage holes for each herb.
3. Prepare Soil: Fill each container with high-quality potting mix, including perlite for improved drainage.
4. Plant: Space the herbs 6-12 inches apart.

5. Water and set: Thoroughly water the containers, then set them in a sunny position.

Container gardening is a versatile and accessible option to cultivate your own herbs, regardless of space or gardening experience. You can have a healthy herb garden right at your doorstep by choosing the perfect containers, preparing the proper soil, and using effective maintenance practices. Embrace the convenience and beauty of container gardening, and enjoy the fresh flavors and health benefits that home-grown herbs provide to your culinary creations.

DESIGNING A MEDICINAL HERB GARDEN

Designing a therapeutic herb garden may be both creative and practical. A well-planned garden not only beautifies your outdoor environment, but it also maximizes the use of the herbs you plant. In this chapter, we'll look at the major components of building a successful medicinal herb garden, such as layout considerations, companion planting, and management methods to help you create a thriving herbal retreat.

Key Elements in Garden Design

Developing an excellent medicinal herb garden necessitates several key elements. Here are some important aspects to keep in mind:

1: Location

- Sunlight: Choose an area that gets at least 6-8 hours of sunlight per day. Most therapeutic herbs thrive in bright sunlight, which promotes strong growth and rich flavors.
- Accessibility: Provide simple access for watering, harvesting, and upkeep. A garden near your kitchen may encourage you to use your herbs more frequently.
- Elements Protection: To make your plants' environment more favorable, consider providing protection from high winds, heavy rain, and extreme temperatures.

2. Layout and Design

- Garden Beds: Set up raised beds or dedicated garden plots to designate your herb garden space. Raised beds increase drainage and are easier to maintain.
- walkways: Create walkways between herb rows to improve access and reduce soil compaction. To achieve a natural effect, use gravel, wood chips, or stepping stones.
- Groupings: Arrange herbs according on their height and development tendencies. Taller herbs, like fennel or dill, can be planted in the back, while

shorter herbs, like thyme and chamomile, should be placed in front.

Companion Planting

Companion planting can help your medical herbs grow and stay healthy, as well as provide pest control and increase flavor. Consider these pairings:

- Basil with Tomatoes: Basil enhances tomato flavor while also deterring pests like aphids and whiteflies.
- Chives with Carrots: Chives can help discourage pests that would normally injure carrots, resulting in a peaceful partnership.
- Peppermint with Cabbage: Planting peppermint near cabbage will help deter cabbage moths and other pests.

Soil Preparation

Proper soil preparation is critical to the success of your medicinal herb garden. Here are some key actions to take:

- Soil Testing: Determine whether any amendments are required by testing the pH and nutrient levels of your soil. Most herbs require a pH range of slightly acidic to neutral (6.0-7.0).
- Amendments: Add organic matter like compost or well-rotted manure to boost soil structure and

fertility. This will provide your herbs the nutrition they need to thrive.

Maintenance Practices

Once your herb garden is planted, regular maintenance will assure its durability and productivity:

1: Watering

- consistency: Regular watering is required, especially in the first few weeks after planting. Aim to keep the soil moist but not saturated.
- Mulch: Apply a layer of organic mulch around your herbs to keep them moist, weed-free, and at stable soil temperatures.

2. Pruning and Harvesting

- Regular Harvesting: Frequent harvesting promotes bushier growth and inhibits flowering, which might reduce flavor. To prevent plant damage, use clean scissors or shears.
- Pruning: Remove dead or yellowing leaves on a regular basis to improve ventilation and lower the risk of disease.

Example: Designing a Medicinal Herb Garden

1. Choose Your Location: Find a sunny place in your yard with sufficient drainage.
2. Plan a Layout: Design a rectangular raised bed that is about 4 feet wide and 8 feet long. Plan paths on both sides for convenient access.
3. Select Companion Plants: Consider basil, chives, peppermint, and thyme for their beneficial associations.
4. Prepare the Soil: Test your soil and add compost and organic debris to create a nutrient-dense environment.
5. Begin Planting: Arrange taller herbs in the back and shorter ones in the front, according to your plan.

Designing a therapeutic herb garden is an interesting experience that blends creativity and functionality. By taking into account important factors such as location, layout, companion planting, and care, you can design a beautiful and useful garden that not only enhances your outside space but also supplies you with fresh herbs for health and wellness. Embrace the effort and reap the numerous benefits of growing your own medical herb sanctuary.

COMPANION PLANTING STRATEGIES

Companion planting is a gardening practice in which different plants are intentionally placed together to benefit one other. This time-honored strategy can boost growth, repel pests, and improve the general health of your garden. In this chapter, we'll look at the basic principles of companion planting, effective therapeutic herb tactics, and practical examples to help you construct a thriving and harmonious herbal garden.

Principles of Companion Planting

Companion planting is based on the premise that particular plants can help each other flourish, increase flavor, and repel pests. Understanding the ideas underlying this strategy will allow you to make more informed selections about which herbs to plant together.

1. Mutual Benefits

- Nutrient Sharing: Some plants have deep roots that draw nutrients up from the soil, making them available to their shallow-rooted neighbors.
- Pest Control: Some herbs can repel pests or attract beneficial insects that eat hazardous pests.

2. Plant Compatibility

- Similar Growth Needs: Select plants with comparable sunshine, water, and soil requirements to guarantee they thrive together.
- Growth Habits: To maximize space and light exposure, pair taller plants with shorter ones.

Effective Companion Planting Strategies

Here are some useful ideas for companion planting with medicinal herbs:

1. Plant Pairing for Pest Control.

- Basil and tomato: Basil not only improves the flavor of tomatoes, but it also repels pests like aphids and hornworm. Plant them together for better growth and yield.

- Lavender and Rosemary: Both herbs are drought tolerant and grow under comparable conditions. Lavender repels insects, although rosemary can deter pests such as cabbage moths.

 2. Improving Growth and Flavor

- Chives and carrots: Chives emit sulfur compounds that can prevent carrot flies, and their growth patterns compliment one another in the garden. This combo may result in healthier carrots.

- Mint and cabbage: Mint can assist to prevent cabbage moths and other pests that attack cabbage plants. Just be careful, as mint can grow quickly; try planting it in a container.

3. Attracting Beneficial Insects

- Calendula and Basil: Planting calendula alongside basil plants attracts pollinators and beneficial insects like ladybugs and lacewings, which eat pests like aphids.

- Nasturtiums and other herbs: Nasturtiums are wonderful trap crops that will keep pests away from your therapeutic herbs while bringing pollinators to your yard.

Practical Examples of Companion Planting

Example 1: The Herbal Trio

- Plant Basil, Tomatoes, and Marigolds - Layout: Place basil next to tomatoes and marigolds in between.
- Benefits: Basil improves tomato flavor and repels pests, but marigolds inhibit nematodes and attract pollinators.

Example 2: The Pollinator Garden.

- Ingredients: Lavender, Bee Balm, and Thyme - Layout: To attract a variety of pollinators, plant clusters of lavender, bee balm, and thyme.
- Benefits: Lavender attracts bees and butterflies, and bee balm (Monarda) gives nectar. Thyme can be

used as a ground cover to help prevent weeds and conserve moisture.

Tips for Successful Companion Planting.

- Begin Small: Test out a few companion plant combinations in your garden to see how they work together.
- Observe and Adjust: Pay attention to how plants interact over time, and be prepared to change your arrangement if certain combinations aren't working.
- Keep Records: Keep a gardening notebook to track the effectiveness of your companion plant pairings and improve your planting techniques in the future.

Companion planting can significantly increase the output and health of your medicinal herb garden. Understanding the concepts of plant compatibility and adopting successful matching tactics will help you establish a flourishing garden that not only delivers an abundance of herbs but also promotes a healthy ecology. Embrace companion planting and watch your herbal garden bloom in harmony!

TROUBLESHOOTING COMMON ISSUES

Identifying and Resolving Common Issues

Even the most experienced herbal gardener can encounter difficulties along the road. Identifying and resolving common issues, such as withering leaves, stunted growth, and low yields, is critical for keeping a healthy and productive herbal garden. In this chapter, we'll look at some common concerns, how to diagnose them, and practical ways to get your garden back on track.

Common Problems and Solutions

1. Wilted Leaves

- Symptoms: Leaves droop or look limp.
- Possible Causes: - Underwatering: The soil may be excessively dry.
- Over-watering: Roots could become soggy, inhibiting effective oxygen intake.

- Solutions: - Check soil moisture levels. If it is dry several inches down, water deeply. If the soil is damp, allow it to dry before watering again.

2. Yellowing Leaves

- Symptoms: Yellowing of the leaves, usually

beginning with the oldest.
Possible causes include nutritional deficiency (lack of vital elements such as nitrogen).
- Pests and Diseases: Problems like root rot or aphid infestation.

- Solutions: - Use a balanced organic fertilizer, preferably nitrogen-rich.
- Inspect for pests or symptoms of disease, and take appropriate action if identified.

3. Stunted Growth

- Symptoms: Plants don't develop or create new leaves.
Possible Causes:Poor Soil Quality: The soil may be deficient in nutrients or not well-drained.
- Compression: Roots may have difficulty growing in compacted soil.

- Solutions: - Add organic matter (e.g. compost) to improve soil nutrient content and drainage.
- Gently aerate the soil around the plant roots to promote healthy growth.

Troubleshooting Tips:

- Regular Observation: Spend time in your garden on a regular basis to identify problems early on.
- Keep a Gardening Journal: Record plant health and

changes to spot trends or recurring issues.
- Ask for help: Don't be afraid to ask local gardening organizations or online forums for advice.

PEST AND DISEASE MANAGEMENT

Pests and diseases can be serious hazards to your herbal garden, reducing plant health and productivity. The ability to recognize these hazards and understand how to control them is critical for a successful gardening experience. In this section, we will look at common pests and illnesses, as well as how to identify them and implement effective control measures.

Common Pests and their Management

1. Aphids

- Symptoms: Small, soft-bodied insects appear on new growth; leaves may curl or yellow.
- Management Strategies: - Natural Predators: Introduce ladybugs or lacewings to eat aphids.
- Neem Oil: Spray neem oil to repel aphids while protecting beneficial insects.

2: Whiteflies

- Symptoms: Small, white flying insects swarm on the undersides of leaves, and sticky residue may be

present.
- Management Strategies: - Yellow Sticky Traps:
Capture adult whiteflies using these traps.
- To reduce infestations, spray affected plants with
insecticidal soap.

3. Spider Mites

- Symptoms: Tiny, spider-like pests spin fine webs;
leaves may be mottled or discolored.
- Management Strategies: - Water Spray: Spray
afflicted plants with water to remove mites.
- Miticides: Use organic miticides if the infection
persists.

Common Diseases and Management

1. Powdery Mildew

- Symptoms: White, powdery patches on leaves and
reduced growth.
- Management Strategies: - Improve Air Circulation:
Properly space plants for optimal airflow.
- Fungicidal Sprays: Apply organic fungicides to the
affected regions.

2: Root Rot

- Symptoms include wilting plants, discolored roots,
and a bad odor.

- Management Strategies: - Soil Drainage: Maintain appropriate drainage to avoid overwatering.
- Remove Affected Plants: Diseased plants should be uprooted and disposed of to avoid spread.

3: Leaf Spot

- Symptoms: Dark blotches on the leaves, usually with yellow halos.
Management Strategies:Remove Affected Leaves: Prune any leaves that exhibit symptoms to avoid further spread.
- Fungicide Application: Use organic fungicides as a precaution.

Understanding the common difficulties, pests, and illnesses that might impact your herbal garden will allow you to take preventative actions and respond efficiently when problems develop. Remember that each garden is unique, so what works for one may not work for another. Stay vigilant, patient, and enjoy the process of cultivating your herbal refuge!

Soil Health and Fertility Concerns

A healthy soil is the foundation of a successful herb garden. It not only supplies vital nutrients, but it also promotes healthy root systems and good microbial life. However, soil health and fertility can deteriorate with time owing to a variety of reasons, resulting in low plant growth and output. In this section, we'll look at typical soil health issues and practical ways to repair and maintain soil fertility.

Common Soil Health Issues:

1. Compacted Soil

- Symptoms include poor drainage, stunted plant development, and difficulty digging.
- Causes: High foot traffic, overtilling, or a lack of organic matter.

- Solutions: - Aeration: Use a garden fork or aerator to break up compacted soil.
- Organic Matter Addition: Use compost or well-rotted manure to increase soil structure and nutrient availability.

2. Nutritional Deficiency

- Symptoms include yellowing leaves, reduced development, and poor flowering or fruiting.
- Causes: Inadequate soil nutrients from leaching or poor soil management.

- Solutions: - Soil Testing: Perform a soil test to assess nutrient levels and pH.
- Fertilisation: To treat specific shortages, use organic fertilizers such as bone meal (phosphorus)

and fish emulsion (nitrogen).

 3. pH Imbalance

- Symptoms include poor growth, fading leaves, and nutrient shortages.
- The causes are: Soil can become overly acidic or alkaline, limiting nutrient availability.

- Solutions: - Adjusting pH: - Add lime to increase pH and decrease acidity.
- Use sulfur or organic debris to reduce pH (raise acidity).
- Re-test Soil: After making modifications, re-test the soil pH to confirm it is within the appropriate range (most herbs require 6.0 to 7.0).

Tips to Maintain Soil Health

- Crop Rotation: Rotate your herbs every year to avoid nutrient deficiency and soil-borne illnesses.
- Cover Crops: Plant cover crops in the off-season to improve soil structure and reduce erosion.
- Mulching: Use organic mulch to control weeds, conserve moisture, and gradually improve soil fertility as it decomposes.

SEASONAL CHALLENGES & SOLUTIONS

Every season presents distinct problems and

opportunities for your herbal garden. Understanding how seasonal variations influence your plants allows you to predict problems and apply effective solutions. In this part, we'll look at common seasonal issues and offer practical advice to help you handle them.

Seasonal challenges

1: Spring Frost

- Symptoms: Unexpected cold temperatures harm or kill new growth.
Solutions: - Cover fragile plants with frost cloths or blankets during chilly nights.
- Transplant Timing: Defer transplanting until after the final projected frost date.

2. Summer Heat

- Symptoms include wilting plants, leaf burn, and lower yields.
Solutions: Mulching: Use a thick layer of mulch to keep soil moist and regulate temperature.
- Watering Schedule: Water in the early morning or late evening to reduce evaporation.

3: Autumn Rains

- Symptoms: Excessive moisture in the soil, higher

risk of root rot and fungal diseases.
- Solutions: - Well-Drained Soil: Keep garden beds well-drained to avoid waterlogging.
- Harvesting Early: If heavy rains are expected, plan to harvest herbs early.

Tips for Seasonal Success

- Plan Ahead: Create a seasonal gardening calendar to keep track of crucial tasks such as planting and harvesting periods.
- Observe Weather Patterns: Pay attention to local weather forecasts and adjust your gardening techniques accordingly.
- Remain Flexible: Be prepared to adapt your care procedures in response to changing weather conditions.

Understanding soil health and the seasonal challenges of gardening will help you better care for your herbal garden. Remember that gardening is a learning process; try with various ways to see what works best for your specific environment.

EXPANDING YOUR HERBAL KNOWLEDGE

As you begin your adventure of producing and using therapeutic herbs, the pursuit of information will be a lifetime activity. Whether you want to learn more about herbal practices, network with like-minded people, or embrace sustainable habits for the future, growing your herbal knowledge may be both educational and fulfilling. In this chapter, we will look at many resources, communities, and practices to help you continue your herbal journey.

Resources for Further Learning

Books and Publications

- Herbal Text: To expand your knowledge, read traditional herbal works as well as recent guidelines.

- Magazines and journals: To stay up to date on the newest research and practices in herbal medicine, subscribe to herbal magazines such as Herb Quarterly or academic journals that specialize in it.

Online Resources

- Websites: Use trustworthy herbalism websites like American Herbalists

- Online Courses: Consider taking online courses or webinars that cover all elements of herbal therapy, from basic botany to advanced formulation methods.

Local Library and Botanical Gardens

- Library Resource: Make use of local libraries, which frequently offer collections of herbal books and resources. Many also provide courses or talks on herbal themes.

- Botanical Gardens: Botanical gardens offer classes and guided tours that focus on medicinal plants. They frequently provide useful information on plant care and usage.

Connecting with Herbal Communities.

Local Herbalists and Workshops

- Herbal Meet-ups: Attend local herbal workshops or gatherings to meet practitioners and gain hands-on experience. These events might be found on community boards or in social media groups.

- Herbal Guilds: Join a local or national herbalist guild, which frequently organizes events, classes, and networking opportunities.

Online Communities

- Social media groups: Join herbalism-related Facebook groups and Instagram pages. Participating in online groups can bring encouragement, inspiration, and shared information.

• Forums & Discussion Boards: Participate in forums like the Herbal Remedies Forum to ask questions, exchange experiences, and learn from others.

Networking.

• Conferences and Events: Attend herbal conferences to meet fellow herbalists, learn from specialists, and broaden your knowledge. Look for events such as the International Herb Symposium and local herb festivals.

CONTINUING YOUR HERBAL JOURNEY

Lifelong Learning

• Workshops and Classes: Seek for workshops that cover advanced herbal topics, such as herbal formulation or foraging techniques.

- Mentorship: Look for a mentor in the herbal community who can offer advice and insight as you build your talents.

Experimentation

- Hands-on Practice: Try various herbs, make your own tinctures or salves, and keep a gardening journal to document your improvement.

- Documentation: Keep a record of your herbal journey, including successful practices, problems, and the effects of different herbs on health and wellness.

Setting Goals

- Personal Goals: Determine short- and long-term objectives for your herbal practice. This could include growing your herb garden, learning new preparation techniques, or deepening your understanding of a particular plant.

SUSTAINABLE HERBAL PRACTICES FOR THE FUTURE

Ethical Sourcing

- Wildcrafting Responsibly: When foraging for wild herbs, practice sustainable wildcrafting by taking only what is necessary and allowing plants to regrow.

- Supporting Local Growers Whenever feasible, buy herbs from local organic farms or herbal businesses that value sustainability.

Environmentally Friendly Gardening

- Organic Practice: Composting, natural pest management, and crop rotation are examples of organic gardening approaches that can help to improve soil health and biodiversity.

- Water Conservation: Use rainwater gathering and smart irrigation techniques to save water in your herb garden.

Advocacy and Awareness.

- Herbal education: Share your knowledge with your friends and family to raise awareness about the benefits of herbal medicine and ecological practices.

- Community Involvement: Get involved in local projects that promote environmental sustainability and medicinal plant conservation.

Expanding your herbal knowledge is a rewarding journey that can significantly improve your experience as a herbal gardener and practitioner. By investigating resources, interacting with communities, and committing to sustainable practices, you can gain a better understanding of herbalism while also benefiting the environment and society. Continue learning, sharing, and growing!

www.ingramcontent.com/pod-product-compliance
Lightning Source LLC
Chambersburg PA
CBHW051607250726

48653CB00004BA/1385

9 798333 609708